Intubating the Critically Ill Patient

Rachel Garvin
Editor

Intubating the Critically Ill Patient

A Step-by-Step Guide for Success in the ED and ICU

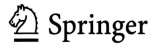 Springer

Editor
Rachel Garvin
Departments of Neurosurgery
Emergency Medicine and Neurology
UT Health San Antonio
San Antonio, TX
USA

ISBN 978-3-030-56812-2   ISBN 978-3-030-56813-9   (eBook)
https://doi.org/10.1007/978-3-030-56813-9

This Springer imprint is published by the registered company Springer Nature Switzerland AG
The registered company address is: Gewerbestrasse 11, 6330 Cham, Switzerland

For years my dad said "you should write a book." He never really said what about, and I don't think specific content mattered so much. It was more along the lines of what I could teach to others. When he learned of the plans for this publication he was so excited, in his own earnest, pragmatic, and understated way. He would have been so proud to have seen this come to fruition but unfortunately died during the writing process. Despite my best efforts, I watched his dignity, mental and physical strength get stripped during a prolonged hospital stay. He remained stoic throughout, a testament to his steadfast nature. My love of attention to detail and analytical thinking are gifts from him that I hope elevate the level of information presented in this book and enhance the knowledge of those that care for the sickest patients. Treat each patient in the same manner that you would want your loved one to be treated. One size does not fit all. Thanks Dad.

Rachel Garvin

Preface

There are many books available on how to pass an ETT through the cords. But what about the preparation needed beforehand? During my years of practice, I have witnessed intubations gone awry because of no preparation and no plan **B.** No two airways are alike, and the tools that we use to help us predict airway difficulty are not 100%.

Plan for Success but Prepare for Failure. This is the motto that I go by for every single airway. It is what I have taught my fellows, residents, advanced practice providers, and students as well. There have been many times I have gone to plan C, but in a controlled and calm manner with all team members doing their part because they all knew the plan.

Without an airway, you have pretty much nothing. Why not make sure we are doing right by our patients every time? This book looks at the who, what, where, when, and how of airway management. Everything up until placing the tube between the cords. Everything up until that point is the most important part of airway management. From the ED to the ICU, be the master of airway preparation and execution. Remember, patients are not protocols. Every situation is unique. Plan for success, but prepare for failure.

San Antonio, TX, USA   Rachel Garvin, MD, FNCS

Acknowledgments

Thank you to all my colleagues that took the time to prepare these chapters. Despite hectic schedules and busy lives, you all are an incredible group of practitioners, dedicated to outstanding patient care.

A huge thank you to my husband, Dan, my daughters, Zoe and Emma, and my boys Milo LL Cool J and Sir Charles von Biscuit who encouraged me every step of the way.

In memory of my father, Dr. Stanley G. Siegel, who always knew I would publish a book one day.

Contents

Contributors

Colleen Barthol, PharmD Department of Pharmacotherapy & Pharmacy Services, University Health System, San Antonio, TX, USA

Jordan B. Bonomo, MD, FCCM, FNCS Department of Emergency Medicine, University of Cincinnati College of Medicine, Cincinnati, OH, USA

Bradley A. Dengler, MD Department of Neurosurgery, Walter Reed National Military Medical Center, Bethesda, MD, USA

Amanda L. Fowler, PharmD, BCPS Department of Pharmacotherapy and Pharmacy Services, University Health System, San Antonio, TX, USA

Shaheryar Hafeez, MD Department of Neurosurgery, UT Health San Antonio, San Antonio, TX, USA

Zachary Kendrick, MD Department of Emergency Medicine, UT Health San Antonio, San Antonio, TX, USA

Georgia J. McRoy, MD Department of Emergency Medicine, UT Health San Antonio, San Antonio, TX, USA

Adriana Povlow, MD Department of Emergency Medicine, UT Health San Antonio, San Antonio, TX, USA

Denise M. Rios, MSN, RN, ACNP-BC Department of Neurosurgery, UT Health San Antonio, San Antonio, TX, USA

Rahul K. Shah, MD Department of Neurology/Neuro Critical Care, Bakersfield Memorial Hospital, Bakersfield, CA, USA

Jessica Solis-McCarthy, MD Department of Emergency Medicine, UT Health San Antonio, San Antonio, TX, USA

Danielle R. Stevens, MD Department of Emergency Medicine, UT Health San Antonio, San Antonio, TX, USA

Chapter 1
Who Needs Intubation?

Georgia J. McRoy

Key Points
- Endotracheal intubation is an invasive procedure.
- Understanding the clinical scenarios requiring advanced airway management is essential to critical care management of patients.
- Common indications for intubation are the following:
  - Failure to ventilate.
  - Failure to oxygenate.
  - Airway protection.
  - Expected clinical course.
  - Airway obstruction.
- Both hypoxemia and hypercapnia can lead to respiratory arrest and cardiovascular collapse.

G. J. McRoy (✉)
Department of Emergency Medicine, UT Health San Antonio, San Antonio, TX, USA

© Springer Nature Switzerland AG 2021   1
R. Garvin (ed.), *Intubating the Critically Ill Patient*,
https://doi.org/10.1007/978-3-030-56813-9_1

Failure to Ventilate: Hypercapneic Respiratory Failure

- Unlike oxygenation which is a passive process, ventilation is an active process.
- Obstructive diseases such as asthma and COPD can result in CO_2 retention [1, 6, 7, 11].
- These patients also develop bronchoconstriction and airway inflammation.
- Other causes of hypercapnia include the following [9, 10]:
  - Metabolic (dehydration, malnutrition).
  - Muscular weakness (from neuromuscular diseases or spinal cord injury).
  - Drug-induced hypopnea [6, 9, 11].
      Alcohols, barbiturates, opiates, benzodiazepines, antidepressants, sedatives-hypnotics, stimulants.
  - Over sedation.
- For an acute respiratory acidosis, PCO_2 does not have to be very high to cause altered mental status [10, 13].
- Patients with chronic obstructive lung diseases can have acute on chronic respiratory acidosis. These patients can have very high PCO_2, but because of chronic retention can tolerate better (look for a high bicarbonate on your chemistry or significant base excess on your blood gas).
- Patients with retention of CO_2 and not responding to interventions such as CPAP, BIPAP may need intubation if noninvasive methods fail [1, 5].
- *Don't let the numbers fool you!* There can be a state of respiratory acidosis in setting of uncompensated metabolic acidosis even with a $paCO_2$ that is within normal range.
- Acute primary respiratory acidemias have a *direct inverse relationship between pH and pCo2*:
  - pH 7.30 →pCO_2 50
  - pH 7.20→ pCO_2 60
  - pH 7.1 → pCO_2 70
- If the numbers do not directly inversely match, there is a second process going on.

Failure to Oxygenate: Hypoxemic Respiratory Failure

- Oxygenation is a passive process and gets altered by mechanisms that interrupt diffusion.
  - Causes of failure to oxygenate: Problem with V/Q mismatch.
      Pneumonia and other secretions [1].
      - Alveoli gets full of material that impedes oxygen diffusion.
      Pulmonary edema/effusion [1, 6, 15].
      - Interstitial fluid and fluid compressing lung tissue prevents diffusion.
      Pneumothorax or other collapse (atelectasis) [3, 4, 8].
      - Collapsed lung cannot diffuse oxygen.
      Pulmonary embolism [6, 8].
      - No blood flow, no place for O_2 to diffuse to.
      Poisons (cyanide).
      - Does not allow oxygen to be used.
  - Patients with progressively worsening hypoxia often become distressed and agitated before becoming cyanotic [1, 3, 9, 15].
  - Hypoxia can lead to deterioration of mental status to the point of obtundation [1, 9, 13].
  - Hypoxia can lead to respiratory arrest and cardiovascular collapse [5].
  - *Be wary of the sick agitated patient – this could be hypoxia and sedating them could lead to devastating consequences!* [3]
  - If possible, a definitive airway should be placed before the situation becomes emergent.
  - Some patients can become hypoxemic and develop respiratory failure just from their work of breathing [5].
  - Asthmatics can have both a failure to oxygenate and a failure to ventilate due to secretions and bronchoconstriction [3, 6, 7].

- Sepsis causes an increased oxygen consumption coupled with a decreased oxygen delivery which affects the body's ability to properly oxygenate and fulfill all of its metabolic needs [6, 10, 11].
- In these patients, airway management can become a necessity to help the body deal with metabolic acidosis but requires appropriate ventilator settings to achieve compensation [6, 10].
- Laboratory values that should give a high index of suspicion for the need to intubate are $PaO_2 < 60$ mmHg and oxygen saturation <90% despite noninvasive interventions [7].

Airway Protection

- Altered mental status
  - Depression of alertness can subsequently lead to inability to protect the airway [1, 9, 13, 15].
  - The loss of protective airway reflexes, such as cough, requires endotracheal intubation whether it is secondary to a neurological or traumatic injury [1, 3, 4, 6, 15].
  - Altered mental status can be caused by multiple etiologies [3, 9, 10, 15]:
      Brain injury (stroke, trauma).
      Infection (CNS, systemic).
      Medications (prescribed, illegal, toxins).
      Temperature control (heat stroke, hypothermia, and serotonin syndrome) [10].
      Status epilepticus unresponsive to other interventions [3, 6, 9–11].
- Aspiration.
  - Mental status can be intact but large volumes in the oropharynx can compromise airway protection [1, 10].
  - Aspiration risks include [2, 3]:
      Ongoing hematemesis.
      Refractory emesis.
      Inability to manage oral secretions (peritonsillar abscess, angioedema).

Expected Clinical Course

- *Combativeness* [3]
  - Patients who are intoxicated, acutely psychotic or under the influence of substances who are a danger to themselves or others
  - May be needed to allow for a safe workup to rule out life threatening injuries
- *Need for transport*:
  - Patients with a high risk of decompensation during transport [1, 9, 10]
  - Critically ill patient with prolonged transport time [1]
- *Trauma*:
  - High likelihood of deterioration [10, 14]
  - Immobilized trauma patients (with cervical spine or facial injuries) presenting with hypoxia, decreased GCS (glascow coma scale), or blood in the oropharynx [3, 8, 10, 12, 15]
  - Patients with facial wounds who may be unable to handle oral secretions [3, 12].
  - Patients with penetrating neck injury or with an expanding hematoma leading to airway compression [3, 12]
  - Chest injuries such as hemo-/pneumothoraces which cause hypoxia despite drainage or proper oxygen therapy, bilateral flail segments or multiple rib fractures resulting in fatigue due to painful respirations [3, 4]

Airway Obstruction

- Airway edema [4, 12]
  - Obstruction can occur from mouth to subglottic region [4, 10].
  - Airway edema often presents with inspiratory stridor.
  - Diminished stridor should prompt a higher index of suspicious for imminent airway collapse [4].
  - Causes of airway edema can include the following:

Anaphylaxis not responding to medical management: progression can lead to complete airway obstruction.

Epiglottis can cause supraglottic obstruction [15].

Angioedema whether it is a genetic predisposition or secondary to a medication.

Ludwig's Angina can prevent orotracheal tube access.

Smoke inhalation can lead to airway edema which may go unnoticed since it is at the glottic level [1, 11].

– These are situations where your approach will be critical and where considerations such as nasotracheal, awake fiberoptic or surgical airway may need to be considered [2].

- Foreign bodies (FB) [15]
  - Aspirated items can obstruct airway supraglottically, at the glottis or infraglottic, including the trachea [3].
  - History is of the utmost importance, especially in the pediatric population.
  - Maintaining calm and comfort of the patient is vital to prevent further airway compromise.
  - If unable to remove the foreign body, placing a definitive airway and sedating patient to maintain oxygenation until appropriate resources obtained for FB removal.
- Difficult anatomy
  - Anatomical conditions that can contribute to a more difficult airway include the following [2, 3, 6, 8, 11, 12, 15]:
    Poor dentition
    Bull neck
    Obesity
    Orofacial masses
    Macroglossia
    Small mandible
    Restricted mouth opening
    Major burns
    Anterior vocal cords

– Other conditions that can affect the management of airways include the following:
Tracheomalacia
Subglottic stenosis
Mediastinal mass

References

1. Brown C, Walls R, Grayzel J. UpToDate. 2008. In: Uptodate.com. http://www.uptodate.com/contents/the-decision-to-intubate.
2. Bucher J, Cuthbert D. The difficult airway: common errors during intubation – emDOCs.net – emergency medicine education. In: emDOCs.net - Emergency Medicine Education. 2019. http://www.emdocs.net/difficult-airway-common-errors-intubation/.
3. Carley S, Gwinnutt C, Butler J. Rapid sequence induction in the emergency department: a strategy for failure. Emerg Med J. 2002;19:109–13.
4. Divatia J, Bhowmick K. Complications of endotracheal intubation and other airway management procedures. Indian J Anaesth. 2005;49:308–18.
5. Divatia J, Myatra S, Khan P. Tracheal intubation in the ICU: life saving or life threatening? Indian J Anaesth. 2011;55:470.
6. Dufour D, Larose D, Clement S. Rapid sequence intubation in the emergency department. J Emerg Med. 1995;13(5):705–10.
7. Guthrie K. Near fatal asthma. In: Life in the fast lane. 2019. https://lifeinthefastlane.com/acute-severe-asthma/.
8. Ho A, Ho A, Mizubuti G. Tracheal intubation: the proof is in the bevel. J Emerg Med. 2018;55(6):821–6.
9. Hua A, Haight S, Hoffman RS, Manini AF. Endotracheal intubation after acute drug overdoses: incidence, complications, and risk factors. J Emerg Med. 2017;52(1):59–65.
10. Nickson C. Rapid Sequence Intubation (RSI) LITFL CCC Airway. In: Life in the Fast Lane LITFL Medical Blog. 2015. https://litfl.com/rapid-sequence-intubation-rsi/.
11. Reid C, Chan L, Tweeddale M. The who, where, and what of rapid sequence intubation: prospective observational study of emergency RSI outside the operating theatre. Emerg Med J. 2004;21:296–301.

12. Sakles J, Mosier J, Patanwala A, Arcaris B, Dicken J. The utility of the C-MAC as a direct laryngoscope for intubation in the Emergency Department. J Emerg Med. 2016;51(4):349–57.
13. Smith C. Rapid-sequence intubation in adults: indications and concerns. Clin Pulm Med. 2001;8:147–65.
14. Stevenson A, Graham C, Hall R, Korsah P, McGuffie A. Tracheal intubation in the emergency department: the Scottish district hospital perspective. Emerg Med J. 2007;24:394–7.
15. Wang HE, Kupas DF, Greenwood MJ, Pinchalk ME. An algorithmic approach to prehospital airway management. Prehosp Emerg Care. 2005;9(2):145–55.

Chapter 2
When to Pull the Trigger

Zachary Kendrick

> **Key Points**
> - The need for a definitive airway presents on a continuum, from elective to crash.
> - There are factors to help predict how soon a patient may require intubation.
> - Reassessment of the patient is critically important to know which path the patient may be on.
> - Don't rely on the numbers to tell you when to pull the trigger: the clinical evaluation of your patient is the most important; data points only supplement.

Types of Intubation

- *Elective*
  - This is typically done to facilitate a procedure and can be planned out hours to days in advance.

Z. Kendrick (✉)
Department of Emergency Medicine,
UT Health San Antonio, San Antonio, TX, USA
e-mail: KendrickZ@uthscsa.edu

© Springer Nature Switzerland AG 2021
R. Garvin (ed.), *Intubating the Critically Ill Patient*,
https://doi.org/10.1007/978-3-030-56813-9_2

- Not typically done in the Emergency Department, but sometimes in the ICU setting.
    Preparation:
    - Complete history and physical
    - Airway evaluation (LEON) [1]
    - Obtain collateral information
    - Review of allergies
    - Discussion of risks and benefits with patient, guardian, or medical power of attorney
    - Written consent
    - Select delayed versus rapid sequence intubation
    - Select and discuss different sedative and paralytic medications
    - Identify and plan for primary, secondary, and tertiary methods of intubation (direct laryngoscopy, video laryngoscopy, and gum elastic bougie, etc.)

L   Look externally (facial trauma, loose teeth, beard, and large tongue)

E   Evaluate 3-3-2 rule (finger breadths)
        Incisor distance: 3 FB
        Hyoid-mental distance: 3 FB
        Thyroid-to-mouth distance: 2 FB

O   Obstruction (epiglottis, abscess, and trauma)

N   Neck mobility (spinal fusion, cervical spine precautions, and arthritis)

Examples:
- Surgery
    - Nonemergent exam under anesthesia (rigid sigmoidoscopy, esophagogastroduodenoscopy, etc.)
- *Urgent*
    - The patient may have some time before decompensation.
        Preparation:
        - Resuscitate the Patient

- Intubation will be complicated and possibly a terminal procedure unless hemodynamics are carefully optimized, monitored, and protected before, during, and after intubation [2–4].
- Complete history and physical.
- Airway evaluation (LEON) [1]
- Review of allergies.
- Discussion of risks and benefits with patient, guardian, or medical power of attorney.
- Verbal consent if patient has capacity to do so, otherwise consent is implied (unless DNI).
- Select delayed versus rapid sequence intubation.
- Select and discuss different sedative and paralytic medications.
- Identify and plan for primary, secondary, and tertiary methods of intubation (direct laryngoscopy, video laryngoscopy, gum elastic bougie, nasotracheal, and cricothyrotomy, etc.).

Examples include the following:

- Intracranial hemorrhage that is expanding
- Traumatic brain injury with altered level of consciousness
- Pulmonary edema not improving with non-invasive positive pressure ventilation and medications
- Developing acute respiratory distress syndrome (ARDS)
- Smoke inhalation

- *Emergent*
  - The patient is imminently going to lose their airway.
    Preparation:
    - Resuscitate the Patient
      - Resuscitation is still important in the emergent intubation situation.
        Consider rapid crystalloid bolus and/or pressor administration if patient hypotensive [5]. Hyperoxygenate if possible (high flow nasal cannula, BiPAP, etc.) while preparing for intubation - higher PaO_2 will give you more time.

Anticipate initial ventilator setting requirements.

- Adjusting minute ventilation (respiratory rate × tidal volume in L/min) to compensate for acidemic state.
- Adjust PEEP for obstructive processes [6].
- Consider pressure control for restrictive lung pathologies [7–9].
- Consider airway pressure release ventilation (APRV) for severe ARDS [10].

- May not have time for full history and physical.
  - Chief complaint
  - Airway evaluation (LEON) [1]

    Measuring distances with finger breadths may not be feasible in this situation.

    - There may not be enough time.
    - The patient may not be able to participate in the exam.
    - The patient may not tolerate removal of BiPAP/CPAP long enough to allow for evaluation.

    The core concepts of the exam should still be identifiable [11, 12].

    - Abnormalities of neck mobility.
      - Cervical collar in place.
      - Severe arthritis/neck stiffness.
    - Swollen or distorted anatomy.
      - Tongue swelling.
      - Neck hematoma.
      - Neck trauma.
    - Short thyromental distance.
      - "Weak" chin.
    - Abnormal dentition.
      - Dentures.
      - Overbite.
      - Mouth trauma.
- Review of allergies (if known).
- Verbal consent if patient has capacity to do so, otherwise consent is implied (unless DNR/DNI).
- Rapid sequence intubation.

- Choice of sedation/paralytic medications still depends on available history if known.
  - Sedation: based on hemodynamics and indication for intubation.
  - Paralytic: Consider rocuronium if history not known and suspicion high for contraindication to succinylcholine (hyperkalemia, crush injury, significant burn, end-stage renal disease, etc.).
- Identify and plan for primary, secondary, and tertiary methods of intubation (direct laryngoscopy, video laryngoscopy, gum elastic bougie, nasotracheal, and cricothyrotomy, etc.).

  Examples included are the following:
- Anaphylaxis with worsening oropharyngeal edema
- Status epilepticus lasting longer than 30 minutes and refractory to first and second line antiepileptics
- Flash pulmonary edema
- Active, profuse hematemesis

- *Crash*
  - Patient has lost airway or has gone into cardiac arrest.
  - No time for questions but you can bag while you get a plan together.
  - May still require RSI drugs to relax clenched jaw.

Tools to Decide How Much Time You Have

- *Airway Protection* [12]
  - Is the patient clearing their own secretions or are they pooling in the oropharynx?
  - Can they cough (may need to stimulate with suctioning)?
  - Do they have a gag reflex (alone not an indication as some people lack a gag reflex at baseline, but in addition to other factors should be considered higher risk for aspiration)?
  - *Worsening mental status (TBI or stroke).*
- *Work of Breathing* [12]

- Is respiratory fatigue setting in?

  No longer tachypneic, but still with significant metabolic acidosis (no longer compensating)

  Increasing accessory muscle use

  Patient becoming agitated or increasingly anxious
- Is work of breathing not improving with initial interventions?

  Asthma exacerbation refractory to inhaled medications and noninvasive ventilation

- *Rate of Clinical Deterioration* [12]

  Rapidly losing airway: anaphylaxis, epiglottitis, angioedema, trauma with expanding neck hematoma, etc.)

  - A condition that is going to take a long time to resolve (toxic ingestion, angioedema, traumatic brain injury, etc.)
  - Impending cardiac arrest
  - *Venous/arterial blood gas*: NOTE! This is a helpful tool but can be deceiving [11].

    Even if the blood gas looks OK, if the patient is clinically worsening (mental status, work of breathing, rate of deterioration), *intubate. Don't wait for the numbers to tell you what to do!*

    For acidemic patients, make sure that they are appropriately compensated (if you only remember one formula, remember *Winter's Formula*)

    - Bicarb + ½ Bicarb + 8 (+/− 2)
    - Tells you what the Pco_2 should be for compensation in metabolic acidosis

  - Hypoxic versus hypercapnic respiratory failure

    Patient can tolerate hypercapnia longer than hypoxia; there is no compensation for hypoxia!

    Hypercapnia may suggest an urgent intubation whereas hypoxia is usually more emergent.

  - Compensation

    Is patient's breathing pattern compensating for blood gas abnormalities? [12]

    Metabolic acidosis (DKA, sepsis)

  - RESUSCITATE FIRST
  - If patient able to compensate, let them

- If patient begins to tire, consider noninvasive ventilation

  Set a time frame for re-evaluation; i.e., if pH does not improve to >7.2 in 1 hour, move to your next step.
- If noninvasive ventilation fails, *urgent intubation is needed*.

  If setting ventilator rate, set rate high to help with ventilation (20 bpm or higher).

	pH	**CO_2**
Metabolic acidosis	↓	↓
Metabolic alkalosis	↑	↑
Respiratory acidosis	↓	↑
Respiratory alkalosis	↑	↓

	All you need to remember for acid–base disorders in an acute situation
Metabolic acidosis	**$PCO_2 = (HCO_3^-) + (½ HCO3) + 8 +/− 2$ [Winter's formula]**
Acute respiratory acidosis/alkalosis	Direct inverse relationship between pH and pCO_2 7.5/30 ➜ pure respiratory alkalosis 7.3/50 ➜ pure respiratory acidosis

Failure of NIV

- Noninvasive oxygenation/ventilation is an incredibly helpful tool, but knowing when it has failed is critically important.
- Set a time for re-evaluation: NIV will either help to prevent an intubation, or it won't.
- *Has the patient's work of breathing increased* (even if blood gas/spO_2/$etCO_2$ same)?
  - The underlying etiology may be worsening.
  - *Consider an urgent intubation.*

- *Has the patient's work of breathing decreased?*
  - Recheck blood gas, it may be worsening and the patient is going into respiratory failure.
  - *If patient has reached the point of respiratory failure, an emergent intubation should be strongly considered.*
- *Work of breathing is same but blood gas/spO_2/$etCO_2$ is worsening?*
  - The patient may need different settings or may need sedation to allow for better compliance.

    If hypoxic but normocapnic, consider CPAP or high flow over BIPAP.

    If hypercapnic but oxygenating fine, consider BIPAP over high flow NC or CPAP.

    If patient is overly anxious or dyssynchronous with the machine, consider respiratory drive sparing sedation medications.
    - Dexmedetomidine or ketamine are good options.
    - DO NOT use respiratory drive impairing agents such as opioids or repeated doses of benzodiazepines.
  - *While attempting these adjustments, begin preparing for an urgent intubation.*
- *Aspiration risk (abdominal distension)*
  - An inherent disadvantage of a noninvasive ventilation system is that air will inevitably go down the esophagus in addition to the trachea. This can lead to gaseous abdominal distension, vomiting, and create an aspiration risk.
  - Vomiting while wearing a positive pressure mask can be very dangerous as the vomitus is immediately pushed back into the oropharynx and down the trachea.
  - Distention alone should prompt the provider to consider *urgent intubation*. Vomiting, however, should prompt consideration for a more *emergent intubation* scenario to prevent aspiration.

Anticipated Clinical Course [13]

- There are some conditions that despite maximum interventions, you can expect to worsen before they get better.
- Some examples:
  - *Angioedema* [14]

    Epinephrine and antihistamines are of minimal help. Patient needs time for airway swelling to reduce.

    Consider *urgent intubation* if early in swelling, otherwise will become *emergent*.

    Anticipate difficult intubation.
    - Glottic swelling will make normal anticipated endotracheal tube size difficult.
    - Be prepared to use gum elastic bougie and/or perform surgical airway.
  - *Smoke inhalation* [15]

    Patient may appear to be breathing fine, but tracheal burns can cause rapid swelling.

    Securing the airway sooner in an *urgent* manner rather than later in an *emergent* or *crash* manner.

    If unsure, if patient has tracheal burns, consider nasopharyngeal fiberoptic evaluation to look for soot, edema, or other evidence.
  - *TBI/IPH* [16]

    Patient will likely get worse over next 48–72 hours and may need days/weeks/months to improve before they regain ability to protect their own airway.

    Consider *urgent intubation*.
  - *Epiglottitis* [17]
  - *Swelling is going to rapidly obstruct the patient's* airway and will make intubation very difficult.
  - Consider *emergent intubation* to prevent the necessity of a surgical airway situation.
  - *Ludwig's Angina* [17]

    Swelling of the submandibular space that progressively worsens.

    The tongue will be elevated and make intubation difficult and eventually occlude the patient's airway.

    Consider *urgent intubation* before airway is compromised.

References

1. Ji SM, Moon EJ, Kim TJ, Yi JW, Seo H, Lee BJ. Correlation between modified LEMON score and intubation difficulty in adult trauma patients undergoing emergency surgery. World J Emerg Surg. 2018;13:33. Published 2018 Jul 24. https://doi.org/10.1186/s13017-018-0195-0.
2. Jaber S, Jung B, Corne P, et al. An intervention to decrease complications related to endotracheal intubation in the intensive care unit: a prospective, multiple-center study. Intensive Care Med. 2010;36(2):248–55. https://doi.org/10.1007/s00134-009-1717-8.
3. Heffner AC, Swords DS, Neale MN, Jones AE. Incidence and factors associated with cardiac arrest complicating emergency airway management. Resuscitation. 2013;84(11):1500–4. https://doi.org/10.1016/j.resuscitation.2013.07.022.
4. Kim WY, Kwak MK, Ko BS, et al. Factors associated with the occurrence of cardiac arrest after emergency tracheal intubation in the emergency department. PLoS One. 2014;9(11):e112779. Published 2014 Nov 17. https://doi.org/10.1371/journal.pone.0112779.
5. Panchal AR, Satyanarayan A, Bahadir JD, Hays D, Mosier J. Efficacy of bolus-dose phenylephrine for Peri-intubation hypotension. J Emerg Med. 2015;49(4):488–94. https://doi.org/10.1016/j.jemermed.2015.04.033.
6. Reddy RM, Guntupalli KK. Review of ventilatory techniques to optimize mechanical ventilation in acute exacerbation of chronic obstructive pulmonary disease. Int J Chron Obstruct Pulmon Dis. 2007;2(4):441–52.
7. Fernández-Pérez ER, Yilmaz M, Jenad H, et al. Ventilator settings and outcome of respiratory failure in chronic interstitial lung disease. Chest. 2008;133(5):1113–9. https://doi.org/10.1378/chest.07-1481.
8. Gaudry S, Vincent F, Rabbat A, et al. Invasive mechanical ventilation in patients with fibrosing interstitial pneumonia. J Thorac Cardiovasc Surg. 2014;147(1):47–53. https://doi.org/10.1016/j.jtcvs.2013.06.039.
9. Vincent F, Gonzalez F, Do C-H, Clec'h C, Cohen Y. Invasive mechanical ventilation in patients with idiopathic pulmonary fibrosis or idiopathic non-specific interstitial pneumonia. Intern Med Tokyo Jpn. 2011;50:173–4. author reply 175

10. Zhou Y, Jin X, Lv Y, et al. Early application of airway pressure release ventilation may reduce the duration of mechanical ventilation in acute respiratory distress syndrome. Intensive Care Med. 2017;43(11):1648–59. https://doi.org/10.1007/s00134-017-4912-z.
11. Tintinalli JE, Stephan SJ, John MO, Cline DM, Meckler GD. Intubation and Mechanical Ventilation. In: Tintinalli's emergency medicine: a comprehensive study guide, vol. 2016. 8th ed: McGraw Hill Professional. New York. p. 190–1.
12. Brown CA, Walls RM. Airway. In: Rosens emergency medicine: concepts and clinical practice. 8th ed. Philadelphia: Elsevier; 2018. p. 3–22.
13. Strayer RJ. Acid-Base disorders. In: Rosens emergency medicine: concepts and clinical practice. 8th ed. Philadelphia: Elsevier; 2018. p. 1629–35.
14. Tran TP, Muelleman RL. Allergy, hypersensitivity, angioedema, and Anapylaxis. In: Rosens emergency medicine: concepts and clinical practice. 8th ed. Philadelphia: Elsevier; 2018. p. 1553.
15. Nelson LS, Hoffman RS. Inhaled toxins. In: Rosens emergency medicine: concepts and clinical practice. 8th ed. Philadelphia: Elsevier; 2018. p. 2039.
16. Heegaard WG, Biros MH. Head injury. In: Rosens emergency medicine: concepts and clinical practice. 8th ed. Philadelphia: Elsevier; 2018. p. 345.
17. Melio FR, Berge LR. Upper respiratory tract infections. In: Rosens emergency medicine: concepts and clinical practice. 8th ed. Philadelphia: Elsevier; 2018. p. 965–77.

Chapter 3
Preparing Yourself for Intubation

Denise M. Rios

> **Key Points**
> - Airway plans should be based on reason for intubation and perceived difficulty of airway.
> - Plans should be rendered from start to finish.
> - All team members should be aware of your plan.
> - YOU are placing the airway so YOU check all your equipment.

What Information Do You Need to Know?

There are several key questions to ask before placing that blade:

- Reason for intubation: This will often dictate how much preparation time you have.
  - *Hypoxemia: not much time.*
    Depending on the cause, may be emergent or urgent.
  - *Hypercapnia: often can temporize.*
    Frequently can respond to noninvasive ventilating.
  - *Airway obstruction: depends on etiology.*

D. M. Rios (✉)
Department of Neurosurgery,
UT Health San Antonio, San Antonio, TX, USA
e-mail: guerrad@uthscsa.edu

© Springer Nature Switzerland AG 2021
R. Garvin (ed.), *Intubating the Critically Ill Patient*,
https://doi.org/10.1007/978-3-030-56813-9_3

Smoke inhalation may give you more time than a foreign body.
- *Altered mental status: usually not emergent.*
This is not a lung problem so you have time to optimize your situation.
- Any Airway History:
  - If you are able to get any history from the patient on previous intubations, this can be helpful with regard to the level of difficulty.
  - If possible, review records from the operating room or outside hospital intubation.
    MAC 3, grade 1 view,1 attempt is markedly different from MAC 4, grade 4 view, bougie, 3 attempts, 2 providers.
- Drug Plan:
  - Are you going to do rapid sequence intubation (RSI) or delayed sequence intubation?
  - Are there any medications that may be contraindicated in my patient (examples) [1]:
    End-stage renal disease? May want to avoid succinylcholine.
    Neuromuscular disorder? Need to be careful with any neuromuscular blocker.
    Acute myocardial infarction? May want to avoid ketamine.

What Is Your Intubating Device of Choice: One Size Does Not Fit All

Direct Laryngoscopy (DL), [2].
- Direct visualization of airway structures.
- Blades are curved or straight.
- Curved blades (Mac) made to go in vallecula and pull epiglottis out of the way.
- Straight blade (Miller) is good for floppy tongues or floppy epiglottis.
  - Straight blades go under the epiglottis to lift it out of the way.

- DL can be ideal when the patient can be positioned to line up airway axes.
- DL is best for patients with copious oral fluids (emesis, upper GIB, heavy secretions).
- Anterior airways can be brought more posterior with backwards upwards rightwards pressure (BURP).

Video Laryngoscopy (VL): Camera at the end of the blade with transmitted video image [2].

- Indirect view of airway.
- Some images on a separate screen, others have a screen attached to the handle.
- Some VL blades have a more acute curve which allows for easier visualization of an anterior airway.
- Just because you can see the airway, does not mean you can place a tube!
- It is often better to get a grade II view of the cords when using VL if the blade has an acute angle.
  - Grade II view will allow you to more easily drop your tube through the cords.
- Some VL you can use just like DL.
- VL should not be the first choice if fluid in the airway is an issue (blood, emesis, copious secretions) as video visualization will be impaired.

Fiberoptic:

- Scopes can be used orally or nasally for awake intubations.
- Best for nonemergent intubations as their use requires preparation time and patient cooperation.
- Need to have some comfort level with the equipment prior to use.

What Is Your Plan: A, B, and C?

- Know what you will start with, and what you will change to if you do not get a view: Example:
  - "Based on initial evaluation, I will start with MAC 3 and 7.5 tube."

- – "If airway is too anterior, I will ask for BURP."
- – "If I get a grade 3 view, I will ask for the bougie."
- – "If I have difficulty passing the tube, I will size down to a 7.0."
- ALWAYS have a backup plan ready to go.
- Your team should know your backup plan.
- Have a rescue device: if you need to stop and bag.
  - – Set a threshold ahead of time of when you will stop and bag.

    "If O2 sats gets to less than 90%, I will stop and bag."
  - – Letting a patient get hypoxemic because you think you may see cords, may be detrimental.
  - – *Stopping to bag the patient is not a failure.*
  - – An appropriately sized oral airway is essential for bagging the patient – it keeps the tongue from blocking the airway.
  - – *Laryngeal* mask airway (LMA) or other supraglottic devices can be a life-saver for the hard to bag patient.
  - – These *items* should be out in plain sight and ready to go every time.

    No one wants to be searching the airway cart for equipment when sats are 80%.

Prepare Your Equipment

- Before you intubate, you want to confirm and verify that all equipment and instruments are present and in working condition. Trying to intubate a patient with hematemesis and finding your suction does not work is less than ideal.
- Do not rely on other people to ensure your equipment is in working order: *YOU are the one doing the airway, you* do the final check!
  - – *Reliable IV access*: make sure IVs are working before you push drugs. If access is limited, consider an IO.
  - – Prepare induction medications and post--intubation medications and have them drawn up and doses checked.

  – Increase the frequency of vital sign checks: BP, SaO_2, ECG:

    BP cuff should be set to cycle every 2–3 minutes.

    Continuous pulse oximetry should be placed and increase the volume, so it can be heard when the SaO_2 drops.

    Verify and analyze that waveforms for the pulse oximetry and/or arterial line are appropriate [2]

  – BVM connected to high flow oxygen with peep valve.

  – Working suction with a yankauer.

    This is VITAL. Always check that suction is working and have the catheter right next to you, so you can grab it without taking your eyes off the airway.

  – Two tracheal tubes.

    Size you think you need and one size smaller.

    (check cuff prior) 10–20 ml syringe, lubricating gel, stylet, or bougie already inserted.

  – Colorimeter CO_2 detector to confirm placement of ETT.

  – ETT tape or securing device.

Assign Roles

• Part of your preparation is confirming you have what you need when you need it.

• Before drugs are pushed is the time when equipment and appropriate personnel are confirmed to be available and ready if needed.

• Focused attention of the entire team during induction and intubation are associated with fewer errors and increased safety of a successful intubation [3].

• During intubation the entire team should be attentive and actively ready to assist with the intubation process.

  – What is your rescue plan to maintain oxygenation?

  – Do you think you may need a consultant?

  – Is the airway so difficult (obstruction, FB) that chances for success are low?

- **Never be afraid to ask for help; your patient would want you to.**
- When roles are assigned and confirmed, there should be a pause for questions or safety concerns from the team prior to commencing the procedure [3].
- For more details, see Chap. 5.

References

1. Durbin CG, Bell CT, Shilling A. Elective intubation. Respir Care. 2014;59(6):825–47.
2. Sklar M, Detsky M. Emergent airway management of the critically ill patient. Current Opinion in Critical Care. 2019. www.co-criticalcare.com.
3. Morgenstern J.. Emergency airway management Part 3: intubation – the procedure. First 10 EM: when minutes matter... 2017. www.first10em.com.

Chapter 4
Preparing the Patient

Danielle R. Stevens

Key Points
- It is never too early to preoxygenate.
- Position the patient to optimize first-pass success.
- Resuscitate prior to intubation to avoid risk of cardiovascular collapse.
- Metabolic acidosis requires respiratory compensation.

Intubation Is Not Just Scary for You...Talk to Your Patient

- Patients in the ED and ICU face surroundings and procedures that result in varying degrees of discomfort and distress
- Goals [4]:
    - Gain confidence and cooperation of your patient
    - Identify patient's thoughts and feelings regarding the procedure
    - Describe the procedure in a calm and unhurried manner

D. R. Stevens (✉)
Department of Emergency Medicine,
UT Health San Antonio, San Antonio, TX, USA

© Springer Nature Switzerland AG 2021   27
R. Garvin (ed.), *Intubating the Critically Ill Patient*,
https://doi.org/10.1007/978-3-030-56813-9_4

- – Give patients a realistic depiction of the discomfort and unpleasantness that is anticipated
- Obtain informed consent when possible
- Informed consent elements [4]:
  1. Discussion of nature of the procedure with the patient
  2. Discussion of reasonable alternatives to the procedure
  3. Relative risks and benefits
  4. Patient acceptance and agreement with the procedure
- *Implied Consent*: applicable in emergency circumstances when patient is unable to consent and proxy cannot be reached [4]
- *Universal Consent Form*: developed to allow patient to consent to multiple common procedures rather than using individual form for each procedure [4]
- *Healthcare Proxy*: person appointed by patient to make medical decisions in the event that patient is incapacitated or unable to make decisions on their own [4]
- Laws on whether family members have authority to make decisions for incapacitated patients vary by state [4]
- Assume that your patient *can hear you and tell them what you are doing!*

Monitoring

- Continuous telemetry is vital (Fig. 4.1)
- Continuous pulse ox and $ETCO_2$, if available
- Ensure adequate waveforms prior to procedure (SPO_2, arterial line) – do not wait until you push drugs to ask "is that sat of 75% real?"
- Blood pressure cuff set to cycle every 2–3 minutes, especially if there is no arterial line

Access

- Obtain two large bore (18G) IVs to bilateral antecubital (AC) fossas

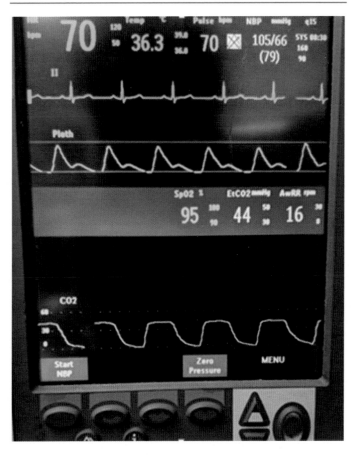

FIG. 4.1 Stevens, Danielle. "Telemetry Monitoring"

- If unable to obtain IV access after two attempts, place IO
- Rule of 2's: 2cc of 2% lidocaine over 2 minutes immediately after placement of IO
- Ensure that all lines flush adequately: You do not want to find out the lines are not functional once you are ready to push drugs!

Preoxygenation

- *Patients breathing room air before RSI can desaturate in 45–60 seconds after sedative/paralytic administration* [11]
- Preoxygenation extends the duration of "safe apnea," that is, time until a patient reaches an O_2 sat of 88–90% [11]
- Mechanism: Denitrogenation. Oxygen washes out nitrogen in the lungs resulting in larger alveolar oxygen reservoir [7]
- Critically ill patients can desaturate immediately
- Patients who are well pre-oxygenated can have periods of "safe apnea" up to 8 minutes [11]
- *Factors That Decrease Safe Apnea Time* [7]
    1. Inadequate Preoxygenation
    2. Airway Occlusion: Leads to loss of functional residual capacity
    3. Pulmonary Shunt: Blood flow to non-oxygenated lung
    4. Increased Oxygen Consumption: Due to high metabolic rate (i.e. sepsis)
    5. Critical Illness
    6. Obesity
    7. Pregnancy
    8. Small Children
- *Apneic oxygenation is not a substitute for effective preoxygenation.*

Tools to Provide Supplemental Oxygen

Oxymask

- *What?* Mask that supplies oxygen up to 40L/min (flush rate oxygen) without requiring a seal (Fig. 4.2)
- *How?* The diffuser mixes oxygen with room air to generate a turbulent flow
- *Who?* Patient with difficulty applying mask and obtaining adequate seal
- *Results?* Mean FeO_2 72% with 69–76% CI [3]

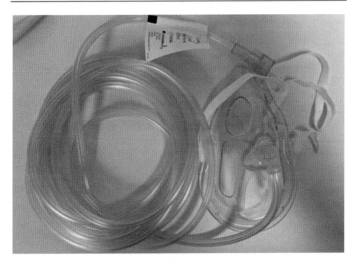

Fɪɢ. 4.2   Stevens, Danielle. "Oxymask"

High Flow Nasal Cannula (HFNC)

- *What?* Heated and humidified high flow nasal cannula
- *How?* Gas is heated to 100% relative humidity at 37° Celsius and can deliver up to 100% FiO_2 at flow rates up to 60 L/min [8]
- *Who?* Anyone who cannot tolerate a mask or requires PEEP (HFNC provides up to 1 mmHg PEEP for each 10L/min of flow in closed mouth breathing) [8]
- *Results?* Role for HFNC remains unclear; Can be helpful if patient cannot tolerate CPAP mask or is at high risk for aspiration

Non-Rebreather Face Mask (NRB)

- *What?* Flush rate oxygen delivered through mask without inspiratory assistance
- *How?* Attached oxygen reservoir bag and one-way valve prevents exhaled air from mixing with oxygen, allows for inspired oxygen concentration of roughly 85% at flow rate of 12–15 L/min [3]

- *Who?* Spontaneously breathing patient, critically ill patients
- *Results?* Mean FeO_2 83% with 80–86% CI, noninferior to bag-valve-mask (BVM) [3]

Bag-Valve-Mask (BVM)

- *What?* Manual resuscitator with non-rebreathing valve
- *How?* BVM and good seal at 15+L/min O_2; Can add PEEP valve to help with alveolar recruitment (Fig. 4.3)
- *Who?* Patients not spontaneously breathing
- *Results?* Mean FeO_2 77% with 73–80% CI [3]
- Caution with BVM as this can lead to regurgitation and aspiration following paralytic administration

Non-Invasive Positive Pressure Ventilation (NIPPV)

- NIPPV such as CPAP or BiPAP use positive pressure via a mask with a tight seal
- Helpful in patients with significant hypoxemia due to atelectasis, hypoventilation or consolidation to obtain highest level of preoxygenation prior to intubation
- Study on obese patients: PPV with CPAP, NIPPV, PEEP valves attached to BVM for 5 minutes, mean SpO_2 98% after preoxygenation and 93% during intubation as compared to 81% in spontaneous breathing group [13]

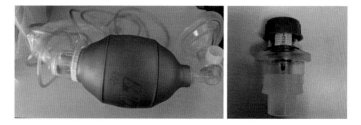

FIG. 4.3 Stevens, Danielle. "Bag-Valve-Mask and PEEP valve"

Apneic Oxygenation

- Oxygenation is a passive process; this can occur even after chemical paralytic given
- Oxygen via nasal cannula at flow rates of 5–60 LPM during intubation provides passive flow [1]
- Significant reduction in incidence of desaturation ($p = 0.002$) and critical desaturation ($p = 0.001$) when apneic oxygenation was implemented [1]
- Significant improvement in first-pass intubation success rate ($p = 0.004$) [1]
- Significant relative risk reduction (RR = 0.76) with apneic oxygenation using low flow oxygen at 15 LPM [1]
- Significant reduction in hypoxemia by 3.04% [1]
- Risk of critical desaturation was halved (RR = 0.51, $p = 0.01$) in trials where apneic oxygenation was employed [1]

Positioning

- Advantages to intubating in upright position: decreased rates of hypoxemia and aspiration [5], longer times to desaturation [3, 6, 9] (Fig. 4.4)
- Preferred in patients with elevated intracranial pressure;
- Can improve glottic view [5]
- Preoxygenation for 3–5 minutes in 20 degrees head up position versus supine position: 386 seconds versus 283 seconds to desaturate from 100% to 95% O$_2$ saturation [6]; 452 seconds versus 364 seconds to desaturate to 93%; 214

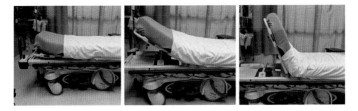

FIG. 4.4 Stevens, Danielle. "Airway Positioning"

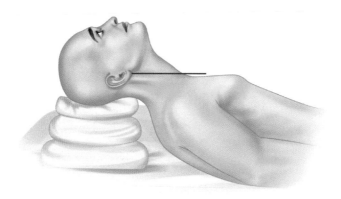

FIG. 4.5 Wilcox, Avi. "Earlobe to sternal notch"

versus 162 seconds to desaturate to 92% in patients with BMI >40 [2]

- Consider reverse trendelenburg position in trauma patients.
- *Earlobe to sternal notch*: Allows appropriate alignment of airway axes (Fig. 4.5)
  - Those axes are oral, pharyngeal, and laryngeal.
  - Without this alignment it is much more difficult to find the cords
- Key maneuvers to relieve obstruction of airway: head elevation, chin lift, jaw thrust
- Avoid cricoid pressure as this can lead to laryngeal or tracheal compression and hinder ventilation

Resuscitation Prior to Intubation

Goals: avoid hypotension, hypoxemia, and metabolic acidosis as all three increase the risk of post-intubation cardiac arrest

- *Hypotension* [10]:
  - Two large bore peripheral IV's; central line not required for short term vasopressors [12]

- Start with fluids but have pressors ready
- Aim for at least normal blood pressure prior to intubation (MAP >65mmHg)
- Decrease dose of sedative to counter drop in venous return and sympathetic tone after IV administration
- Increase dose of paralytic as it may take longer to take effect in shock state
- Increase dose of rocuronium to 1.6 mg/kg as it provides for longer safe apnea time when compared to succinylcholine
- Vasopressors prevent delay in intubation and decrease morbidity and mortality
- Options: push dose vasopressors versus peripheral vasopressor infusions
- Vasopressors can be safely run through peripheral IV for up to 24 hours without risking injury to local tissue (preferably 18g or larger, AC or proximal) [12]
- *Hypoxemia*:
  - Hypoxemia is the enemy; Any PaO_2 you can gain puts the ball more in your court
  - Even for patients that present hypoxemic there are maneuvers that can take an oxygen saturation from 85% to 95% and buy you precious minutes
  - Suction: nasotracheal, orally, nasally; Clearing secretions can dramatically improve oxygenation
- *Delayed-Sequence Intubation*: procedural sedation in order to oxygenate
  - Give 1 mg/kg IV ketamine to allow for adequate pre-oxygenation prior to paralyzing patient for intubation
- Result: increase in O_2 saturation from 89.9% to 98.8% [13]
  - Adequate positioning with patient upright and head elevation as discussed previously
- *Metabolic Acidosis*:
  - These patients are dependent on spontaneous respirations to maintain acid–base homeostasis
  - High risk for acute decompensation peri-intubation if compensation is not maintained

- Before induction place patient on BiPap so that patient is getting assisted breaths with a base pressure support [11]
- Trial of NIPPV during resuscitation efforts may help avoid intubation altogether
- No controlled studies have shown benefit in hemodynamics with bicarbonate infusion, best to correct the underlying problem [11]
- For these critical patients the most experienced person should be at the head of the bed
- Following intubation, ensure the rate of BVM and/or ventilator is appropriate to maintain respiratory compensation
- Obtain serial blood gases to ensure appropriate compensation

References

1. Binks M, Holyoak R, Melhuish T, Vlok R, Bond E, White L. Apneic oxygenation during intubation in the emergency department and during retrieval: a systematic review and meta-analysis. Am J Emerg Med. 2017;35:1542–6.
2. Dixon B, Dixon J, Carden J, Burn A, Schachter L, Playfair J, Laurie C, O'Brien P. Preoxygenation is more effective in the 25° head-up position than in the supine position in severely obese patients. Anesthesiology. 2005;102:1110–5.
3. Driver B, Klein L, Carlson K, Harrington J, Reardon R, Prekker M. Preoxygenation with flush rate oxygen: comparing the non-rebreather mask with the bag-valve mask. Ann Emerg Med. 2018;71:381–6.
4. Hanson W. Chapter 6. Informed Consent and Procedure Documentation | Procedures in Critical Care | AccessAnesthesiology | McGraw-Hill Medical. [online] Accessanesthesiology.mhmedical.com. 2009. Available at: https://accessanesthesiology.mhmedical.com/content.aspx?bookid=414&sectionid=41840230. Accessed 11 Apr 2019.
5. Khandelwal N, Khorsand S, Mitchell S, Joffe A. Head-elevated patient positioning decreases complications of emergent tra-

cheal intubation in the ward and intensive care unit. Anesth Analg. 2016;122:1101–7.

6. Lane S, Saunders D, Schofield A, Padmanabhan R, Hildreth A, Laws D. A prospective, randomised controlled trial comparing the efficacy of pre-oxygenation in the 20° head-up vs supine position*. Anaesthesia. 2005;60:1064–7.

7. Nickson C. Preoxygenation LITFL medical blog CCC airway. In: Life in the Fast Lane LITFL Medical Blog. 2019. https://litfl.com/preoxygenation/. Accessed 11 Apr 2019.

8. Nishimura M. High-flow nasal cannula oxygen therapy in adults. J Intensive Care. 2015; https://doi.org/10.1186/s40560-015-0084-5.

9. Patel A, Nouraei S. Transnasal Humidified Rapid-Insufflation Ventilatory Exchange (THRIVE): a physiological method of increasing apnoea time in patients with difficult airways. Anaesthesia. 2014;70:323–9.

10. Rezaie S. Critical care updates: resuscitation sequence intubation-hypotension kills (Part 1 of 3) – REBEL EM – Emergency Medicine Blog. In: REBEL EM – Emergency Medicine Blog. 2014. https://rebelem.com/critical-care-updates-resuscitationsequence-intubation-hypotension-kills-part-1-of-3/. Accessed 11 Apr 2019

11. Rezaie S. Critical care updates: resuscitation sequence intubation-pH Kills (Part 3 of 3) – REBEL EM – Emergency medicine blog. In: REBEL EM – Emergency Medicine Blog. 2016. https://rebelem.com/?s=pH+kills. Accessed 11 Apr 2019

12. Lewis T, Mercahn C, Altusher D, et al. Safety of the peripheral administration of vasopressor agents. J Intensive Care Med. 2017;34(1):26–33.

13. Turner J, Ellender T, Okonkwo E, Stepsis T, Stevens A, Sembroski E, Eddy C, Perkins A, Cooper D. Feasibility of upright patient positioning and intubation success rates At two academic EDs. Am J Emerg Med. 2017;35:986–92.

Chapter 5
Preparing Your Team

Adriana Povlow

Key Points
- Assigning team roles is vital to ensure a safe, smooth procedure.
- Without roles, chaos often ensues and plans go awry.
- The intubator is the team leader and cannot be shy about speaking up.
- Everyone's role on the team is important to ensure success.

Why Team Preparation Is Necessary?

- Preparing for intubation is akin to a flight crew preparing for takeoff: everyone knows their roles, flight plan is in place with alternate routes if there is turbulence, and if a problem is spotted, nobody is afraid to speak up.
- Arranging the plan for the intubation can take longer than the actual intubation itself, but time spent for preparation

A. Povlow (✉)
Department of Emergency Medicine,
UT Health San Antonio, San Antonio, TX, USA
e-mail: povlow@uthscsa.edu

© Springer Nature Switzerland AG 2021
R. Garvin (ed.), *Intubating the Critically Ill Patient*,
https://doi.org/10.1007/978-3-030-56813-9_5

will save time during the procedure; and may even save a life.

- Everyone loves a good intubation, it can draw a crowd. Crowds can lead to chaos and having control of the room is imperative.
- Even in the face of a chaotic situation, laying out a plan will allow for the most controlled situation possible.

Meet the Members of the Team

You – the intubator:

- The person at the head of the bed holding the laryngoscope calls the shots.
- This is not the time to be shy: the room needs to be controlled by you.
- Let your team know how you want the environment for the procedure.
- Tell the team your plan for the intubation: Plan A, Plan B, and then Plan C.
- *Communicate what information is or is not needed.* Some helpful examples:
  - "Let me know when all drugs are in."
  - "Don't tell me the O_2 sats unless they get below 90%, if they do, then we stop and bag."
  - "Let me know if heart rate and BP are increasing, we may need more sedation."
  - "Let me know if BP is falling and let's have pressors ready to go."
  - "If I need to go to plan C, the crich kit is on the counter."
- Based on the reason your patient needs intubation, your plan should be carefully crafted to ensure all bases are covered and everyone knows how to cover them [1].
- Let team members know they can communicate concerns with you during the procedure. Every team member needs to know their value and that you will listen [1].

The Nurses

- Nurses are the frontline of patient care and are often the only members of your team at some institutions.
- Having the nurses on board with the plan is critical.
- The nurses need to know that they play a crucial role on the team.
- Communicate with nursing early on if you think you may need to intubate. Sometimes assignments need altering to ensure staff are free.
- Clearly convey what is needed to prepare the patient:
  - Are IVs patent?
  - Do we have the drugs/supplies on hand?
- Ask nursing to help assemble team members needed such as respiratory therapy, pharmacy, and X-ray tech.
- Give instructions with closed loop communication for specific medications, route of administration, and dosages.
- Once medications are drawn up, verify that they are correct and ready to go.
- Give your plan for post-intubation sedation. Include specific medications, route of administration, and dosages.

Respiratory Therapist

- You may not always have a respiratory therapist (RT) available, but they can make a big difference in helping the intubation go smoothly.
- A good RT is an invaluable addition to the team.
- Communicate early on when you plan for intubation; this gives the RT time to start gathering supplies and equipment.
- Tell the RT why you are intubating, they may be able to help you select ventilator settings if you are unsure.
- Share your plan for intubation.
- RT can make certain a ventilator is ready to go.
- Other essential items for the RT:
  - BVM with end tidal CO_2 evaluation device.

- PEEP valve.
- Oral airway.
- Oxygen for apneic oxygenation.
- Supplies to secure tube after intubation [1, 2].
- *Communicate with the RT how they can assist you during the procedure*:
  - "If sats get below 90%, please place an oral airway and we will start bagging"
  - "When I see cords I will let you know to hand me the ET tube."

Pharmacist

- Like the RT, you may not always have a pharmacist or pharmacy tech available during an intubation, but they are a great resource for medication selection and preparation.
- Pharmacists may have suggestions on what medications would be best for sedation, paralytics, and post-intubation sedation, based on the patient situation.
- Communicate when you plan to intubate.
- Give instructions with closed loop communication for specific medications, route of administration, and dosage for RSI meds and post-intubation sedation [3].
- Give your plan for post-intubation sedation including specific medication, route of administration, and dosage [3].
- Ensure that medications are appropriately calculated, drawn up and ready to go.

X-Ray Tech

- Once you have your tube in and hear good breath sounds, you need to check placement with a chest X-ray. Your X-ray tech is needed for that!
- Have a team member call X-ray for when your tube is in.

- In critically ill patients, it is good to have them nearby and ready, so you may want to have them called before your tube is in.
- Help your tech position the patient, so you can guarantee an adequate film.
- Make sure you look at your film after it is done: better to not have an unintentional right main stem intubation!

Nursing Technicians/Assistants

- Nursing techs can offer additional support during an intubation.
- Important roles that nursing techs play:
- Ensuring all monitors are precisely hooked up.
  - Making certain oxygen is on the patient correctly.
  - Double checking supplies.
  - Being a support for the patient and family.

References

1. Weingart S. Podcast 92 – EMCrit Intubation Checklist. EMCrit Blog. Published on February 5, 2013. Accessed on January 27th 2020. Available at https://emcrit.org/emcrit/emcrit-intubation-checklist/.
2. Weingart S. Podcast 176 – updated EMCrit rapid sequence intubation checklist. EMCrit Blog. Published on June 27, 2016. Accessed on January 27th 2020. Available at https://emcrit.org/emcrit/intubation-checklist-2-0/.
3. Morgenstern J. Emergency airway management Part 3: intubation – the procedure. First10EM blog, December 11, 2017. Available at: https://first10em.com/intubation/.

Chapter 6
The RSI Potpourri

Amanda L. Fowler

> **Key Points**
> - Rapid sequence intubation (RSI) medications improve intubating conditions, increase success rates, and decrease complications
> - Preinduction medications are a luxury, not a necessity
> - There is no such thing as a "one size fits all" RSI drug
> - *Intubation can hurt… analgesia matters*

Medications for RSI may be divided into three categories:

- Preinduction medications
- Induction medications
- Neuromuscular blocking (NMB) medications

A. L. Fowler (✉)
Department of Pharmacotherapy and Pharmacy Services, University Health System, San Antonio, TX, USA
e-mail: Amanda.Fowler@uhs-sa.com

© Springer Nature Switzerland AG 2021 45
R. Garvin (ed.), *Intubating the Critically Ill Patient*,
https://doi.org/10.1007/978-3-030-56813-9_6

Preinduction Medications

- Used to mitigate physiologic responses to RSI [1–3]
- Efficacy requires administration at least 2–3 minutes prior to induction [1]
  - When utilized, often administered during the preoxygenation phase of RSI [1]
  - *These drugs are not required!*
  - In an emergent situation, patients often do not have the physiologic reserve to support waiting these extra minutes

Preinduction medications [1–3]				
Medication	Dose	Onset	Physiologic benefit	Considerations
Fentanyl	1–3 mcg/kg IV	≤ 30 sec	Blunts sympathetic response to intubation	• May help patients with elevated ICP, hypertensive emergency or myocardial ischemia • Beware loss of sympathetic drive may remove compensatory mechanisms in shock
Atropine	0.02 mg/kg IV	1 min	Counters bradycardia associated with vagal nerve stimulation	• Only recommended in patients with bradycardia or other risk factors for bradycardia • Max single dose 0.5 mg IV
Phenyle-phrine	25–200 mcg IV	<30 sec	Peripheral vasoconstriction	• Only use for patients demonstrating hypotension (not preemptively) • May repeat • Commonly causes reflex bradycardia

- Updates in practice for use of pre-treatment medications [2–5]
  - Lidocaine is no longer recommended due to a paucity of data to support efficacy and side effects (hypotension)
  - Defasciculating doses of noncompetitive NMBs (10% of the paralyzing dose) prior to succinylcholine use are no longer recommended

Evidence for efficacy is limited to a neurosurgical brain tumor patient population

Studies of TBI patients undergoing RSI have not demonstrated benefit

Induction Medications

- There is no such thing as the perfect RSI induction drug; but if there was, it would have....
  - Rapid onset of action
  - Duration equivalent to that of the paralytic used
  - Hemodynamic neutrality
  - Analgesia, sedation, and amnesia
    Remember, intubation and all the procedures that commonly follow, cause pain and discomfort
  - Cerebral protective effects

Induction medications [1–3]

Medication	Dose	Onset	Duration	Physiologic benefit	Considerations
Etomidate	0.3 mg/kg IV (adjusted BW in morbidly obese patients)	10–45 sec	5–15 min	• Hemodynamically neutral • Neuroprotective	• Adrenal suppression. • Myoclonus (in absence of NMB) • No analgesia
Ketamine	1–2 mg/kg IV	30–40 sec	5–10 min	• Analgesia • Hemodynamically positive (increase heart rate and blood pressure) unless catecholamine depleted • Anticonvulsant	• Baseline severe hypertension • Catecholamine depletion • Laryngeal spasm • Acute myocardial infarction • Sialagogue

(continued)

Induction medications [1–3]

Medication	Dose	Onset	Duration	Physiologic benefit	Considerations
Midazolam	0.1–0.3 mg/kg IV or IM	1–5 min (shorter when given with an opioid)	30–80 min	• Amnesia • Anxiolysis • Anticonvulsant	• Hypotension • Paradoxical agitation • Wide dose response variability • Decrease dose when given with an opioid • Reversal agent (flumazenil) available • No analgesia
Propofol	1–2 mg/kg IV (actual BW)	10–45 sec	3–10 min	• Rapid onset and duration • Anticonvulsant	• Hypotension • Bradycardia • Egg & soybean allergy • Lipid emulsion formulation • No analgesia

BW body weight, *IM* intravenous, *IV* intravenous, *NMB* neuromuscular blocker

- Updates in practice for use of induction medications
    - Barbiturate (methohexital) use in the emergency department for RSI has largely been replaced with alternative agents due to drug shortages and risk of hemodynamic instability (similar to propofol) [2]
    - Ketamine sympathomimetic effects can increase intracranial pressures (ICP), but these increases are transient and clinically insignificant; *elevated ICP should not preclude choice of ketamine as an RSI induction medication* [2]
    - Ketamine-induced increased salivation is well-documented; however, routine pretreatment with an anticholinergic (e.g., atropine) is unnecessary [6]
    - Risk of emergence reactions associated with ketamine do not require pretreatment with benzodiazepines [6]

Emergence reactions may be treated effectively with benzodiazepines when they occur

Timely post-intubation sedation (with any sedative) should decrease the likelihood of emergence

Neuromuscular Blocking Medications [1–3, 7]

- Paralysis with NMB medications for RSI has been shown to decrease airway complications and improve first attempt success
- NMBs *do not* confer any analgesia, amnesia, or sedation
  - Every precaution should be taken to avoid paralysis without sedation

    Consideration for the onset and duration of the induction and NMB medications (and any discrepancy thereof) is essential

    Though the onset time of an NMB may exceed that of the chosen induction agent, generally, it is best to routinely administer the induction medication before the NMB to avoid any chance of paralysis without sedation

    Choose and prepare post-intubation sedation medications prior to RSI to minimize time to administration
- When an NMB medication is used, the practitioner must be prepared for the implications of a failed airway
  - Continued bag-valve mask support for the duration of paralysis
  - Use of a supraglottic device
  - Conversion to a surgical airway

- Safety measures should be in place to prevent medication errors with these high-alert medications that halt respiration

Neuromuscular blocking medications [1–3, 7]

Medication	Dose	Onset	Duration	Physiologic benefit	Considerations
Depolarizing NMBs					
Succiny-lcholine	1–2 (1.5) mg/kg IV actual BW	30–60 sec	5–10 min	Shorter duration of action is desirable for patients who require a prompt post-procedure neurologic exam	• Repeated doses not recommended • Hyperkalemia • Increase dose to >2 mg/kg for denervating neuromuscular diseases with an actual or functional decrease in acetylcholine receptors (e.g., myasthenia gravis) • Avoid in known pseudocholine-sterase deficiency due to prolonged paralysis (hours) • Contraindicated for malignant hyperthermia history (personal or family)
Nondepolarizing NMBs					
Rocuronium	0.6–1.2 mg/kg IV	1–2 min (dose dependent)	30–45 min	No effect on serum potassium	• Anticipated difficulty bag-mask ventilating (longer paralysis duration) • Not recommended in disease states with upregulated acetylcholine receptors (i.e., Lambert-Eaton myasthenic syndrome)

Neuromuscular blocking medications [1–3, 7]					
Medication	Dose	Onset	Duration	Physiologic benefit	Considerations
Vecuronium	0.1–0.2 mg/kg IV	2–4 min	20–60 min	No effect on serum potassium	• Anticipated difficulty bag-mask ventilating (longer paralysis duration) • Not generally used for RSI in the absence of drug shortages due to longer onset and duration of action

BW body weight, *IV* intravenous, *NMB* neuromuscular blocker

- Succinylcholine-induced hyperkalemia [2, 7]
  - The average increase in serum potassium after succinylcholine administration is ~0.5 mEq/L (clinically insignificant in most patients)
    Reasonable to avoid in certain populations (renal failure, patients presenting with symptomatic hyperkalemia, etc.)
  - Exaggerated potassium release (increase by 5–15 mEq/L) may occur with prolonged immobilization (critically ill ICU patients), and burn, crush, or denervation injuries approximately 5 days after the injury occurred
- Nondepolarizing NMB reversal with sugammadex [8]
  - Sugammadex is approved for neuromuscular blockade reversal of rocuronium and vecuronium in patients undergoing surgery at 2, 4, or 16 mg/kg actual body weight IV
  - Since RSI indications in the emergency department and ICU are generally emergent (not elective) reversal of iatrogenic paralysis does not remove the indication for a secure airway
    Given the high cost and elimination of the ability to use rocuronium and vecuronium as medications for future intubations in the next 5 minutes to 24 hours (depending on sugammadex dose used), sugammadex use has not been widely adopted in the emergency department

References

1. Mace SE. Challenges and advances in intubation: rapid sequence intubation. Emerg Med Clin N Am. 2008;26:1043–68.
2. Stollings JL, Diedrich DA, Oyen LJ, Brown DR. Rapid-sequence intubation: a review of the process and considerations when choosing medications. Ann Pharmacother. 2014;48(1):62–76.
3. Mason MA, Weant KA, Baker SN. Rapid sequence intubation medication therapies: a review in light of recent drug shortages. Adv Emerg Nurs J. 2013;35(1):16–25.
4. Clancy M, Halford S, Walls R, Murphy M. In patients with head injuries who undergo rapid sequence intubation using succinyl-choline, does pretreatment with a competitive neuromuscular blocking agent improve outcome? A literature review. Emerg Med J. 2001;18:373–5.
5. Kramer N, Lebowitz D, Walsh M, Ganti L. Rapid sequence intubation in traumatic brain injured adults. Cureus. 2018;10(4):e2530. https://doi.org/10.7759/cureus.2530.
6. Green SM, Roback MG, Kennedy RM, Krauss B. Clinical practice guideline for emergency department ketamine dissociative sedation: 2011 update. Ann Emerg Med. 2011;57(5):449–61.
7. Hampton JP. Rapid-sequence intubation and the role of the emergency department pharmacist. Am J Health-Syst Pharm. 2011;68:1320–30.
8. Bridion (sugammadex) [prescribing information]. Whitehouse Station, NJ; Merck & Co, Inc: December 2018.

Chapter 7
Should You RSI?

Jessica Solis-McCarthy

> **Key Points**
> - Certain patients and physiologic conditions make awake intubation a safer choice.
> - Awake intubation requires considerable time and preparation.
> - Goal is to maintain patient's work of breathing.
> - Appropriate anesthesia or sedation monotherapy and a cooperative patient are required.
> - Options for equipment include fiberscopes, rigid laryngoscopes, and laryngeal mask airways (LMAs).
> - Failure to plan for possible failure will lead to catastrophic results.

Why Is RSI Not For Everyone?

- Rapid sequence intubation (RSI) involves giving an induction agent followed immediately by a neuromuscular blocking agent to facilitate endotracheal tube (ETT) placement.

J. Solis-McCarthy (✉)
Department of Emergency Medicine,
UT Health San Antonio, San Antonio, TX, USA
e-mail: SolisJ4@uthscsa.edu

© Springer Nature Switzerland AG 2021
R. Garvin (ed.), *Intubating the Critically Ill Patient*,
https://doi.org/10.1007/978-3-030-56813-9_7

- RSI may not be needed for patients in cardiac or respiratory arrest as these patients may be intubated without pharmacological assistance.
- RSI may also not be the method of choice for those airways that are considered to be difficult.
- Patients may have significant airway obstruction or may be compensating for a physiologic process and RSI can lead the practitioner down the path of the dreaded "can't intubate, can't ventilate" scenario.
- Emergent evaluation and management of critically ill patients with difficult airways often involve significant time constraints, less-than ideal conditions, and unpredictable events that make it impossible to thoroughly evaluate such patients prior to RSI [1, 2].
- A difficult airway may be an unexpected finding.
- ETT placement may be impossible as a result of pathology at the base of the tongue and epiglottis which external assessments will not predict [3].

Are We Afraid Of Awake Intubation?

- Much of the data for the use and success of awake endotracheal intubation come from anesthesia research in a controlled operating room setting.
- In a retrospective study over a period of 12 years, of the 146,252 surgical cases requiring ETT placement, awake intubation took place in only 1.06% of cases. The low percentage trend remained relatively the same throughout the 12 years despite the introduction of video laryngoscopy [4].
- The low frequency of awake intubations is echoed in a smaller 1-year prospective study in the academic emergency setting where out of 456 intubations, 50 were deemed difficult, and only 7 (1.5%) underwent awake intubation [5].
- Given the rarity of such limited clinical indications leading to awake intubations and the lack of frequent medical practice, many feel reluctant to perform the procedure.

- It has been noted in research that when it comes to choosing between RSI and awake intubations, many practitioners lean toward performing RSI, as this is a more familiar technique and is considered to be safer, and more likely to be successful [6, 7].
- In addition to deficiencies in training and experiences in performing awake intubation, other concerns include patient's comfort as well as the significant time investment required for preparation and completion of the procedure.
- Awake intubation allows for a controlled and deliberate evaluation of the posterior pharynx, larynx, supraglottic, and subglottic structures without compromising hemodynamics or level of consciousness.
- If properly planned, awake intubation is not daunting. Planning begins by considering who would make a good candidate as well as timing the preparation and procedure appropriately.
- *If you can do a nasopharyngeal (NP) scope, you can do an awake intubation!*

Who Is A Good Candidate For Awake Intubation?

- A standard definition of a difficult airway is difficult to define in the literature and comes down to the interaction between multiple complex elements including patient factors, clinical settings, and the skills of the practitioner.
- Overall, awake intubation is the preferred method of intubation if
  - the patient is anticipated to be a difficult intubation which may require multiple attempts despite optimized conditions.
  - face mask ventilation or supraglottic devices ventilation are also predicted to be difficult.
  - the risk of "can't oxygenate, can't ventilate" is high [8].

- Ideally, the patient should be cooperative and be consentable.
- Poor candidates include the pediatric patient, adults with cognitive impairment, brain or cervical spine injury, baseline hypoxemia, compensated hypercapnia, hemodynamic instability, and agitation.

Can You Emergently Perform An Awake Intubation?

- Awake intubation is more appropriate for the elective or urgent as opposed to emergent airway.
- In a retrospective study reviewing intraoperative records at an academic center evaluating the amount of time needed to perform an awake intubation in the anticipated difficult airway, *the median time to intubation was 24 minutes* [12].
- The time it took to perform an awake intubation including topicalization added an average of 8 additional minutes onto the total time from entry into the operating room to intubation.
- For each increase in Body Mass Index of 1 kg/m^2, the time to awake intubation increased about 7 seconds [12]
- Although there are published techniques on performing awake intubation using mono therapy without a paralytic, with or without the addition of topical anesthesia, there is no clear evidence supporting the uses of these techniques [9–11]. These mono therapy methods will be discussed further under the "Sedation" section.
- In addition to time, the other limiting factor is whether the necessary equipment is accessible to the practitioner.
- Temporizing measures such as high flow nasal cannula, non-invasive positive pressure ventilation, assisted face mask ventilation, or placement of a supraglottic devices can help in managing an underlying condition to the point when additional expertise or equipment may be available.

- If endotracheal intubation cannot be avoided, creating a decision pathway with multiple options for how to proceed in case of failed plans will help in streamlining airway management.

Preparation: Preoxygenation and Positioning

- As with RSI, appropriate patient positioning and preoxygenation is fundamental in maximizing success.
- *Even though the patient is spontaneously breathing, the higher the PaO2, the more time you will have.*
  - Desaturations with apnea can be further postponed if pre-oxygenation is performed while the patient is in the semi-fowler or high-fowler position or in reverse Trendelenburg.
- Apneic oxygenation via nasopharyngeal catheter or nasal cannula may also be beneficial during the attempted endotracheal intubation [13–17].

Medicating or Steps For Medicating

Step 1: Premedication

Premedicating with anti-sialagogues should be performed as soon as possible to allow time for their desiccating effects.

- An anti-sialagogue is prudent prior to application of topical airway anesthesia to help in decreasing airway secretions and facilitate anesthetic absorption via the mucous membranes (Table 7.1).
- Intravenous *glycopyrrolate* is a quaternary ammonium compound that does not cross the blood-brain barrier and does not cause sedation.
- At a dose of 0.1–0.2 mg, glycopyrrolate has an onset time of 1–4 minutes and duration effects of up to 2–4 h. Some of the rare side effects that can occur from glycopyrrolate use include cardiac arrhythmias, urinary retention, relaxation of lower esophageal sphincter, mydriasis, and cycloplegia.

TABLE 7.1 Information on anti-sialagogues [20]

Anti-sialagogues	Time of onset	Duration	Side effects	Max dose
Glycopyrrolate	1 min	IV: 7 hours	Cardiac arrhythmias, flushing, vomiting, urinary retention, nasal congestion	IV: 4 mcg/kg
Atropine	30 minutes	4 hours	Tachycardia, drowsiness	IV: 0.4–1 mg

- *Atropine* is another anti-sialagogue that is commonly utilized. However, as a tertiary amine it can cross the blood-brain barrier leading to hemodynamic effects such as tachycardia and increased drowsiness [15, 17–19].

Step 2: Topical Anesthesia

Topical anesthesia is paramount when performing awake laryngoscopy as this will help with maximizing patient comfort, blunt reflexes that comes with direct manipulation of the highly innervated upper airway structures and limit the need to supplement with any sedative medications such as opiates or benzodiazepines.

- Depending on the approach for awake intubation, *topical anesthesia* can be broken down into the respective areas: *nasal cavity* and *nasopharynx*, *oral cavity* and *oropharynx*, and *larynx above and below the vocal cords*.
- Anesthetics commonly utilized include *lidocaine* and *cocaine*; however, the choice of which to use comes down to availability and contraindications.

Nasal Cavity and Nasopharynx

- For the nasal vasoconstriction and anesthetic part of the procedure, a variety pieces of equipment will be needed (see Fig. 7.1).

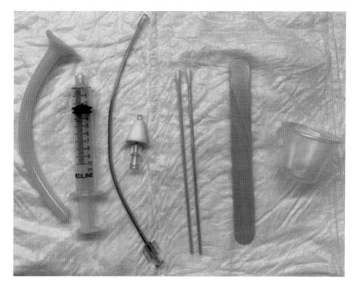

Fig. 7.1 Equipment needed for nasopharyngeal vasoconstriction and nasopharyngeal/oropharngeal anesthesia: Nasopharyngeal airway, 10 mL syringe, atomizers such as LMA MADgic® laryngotracheal mucosal atomization device and MAD intranasal mucosal atomization device, cotton-tip applicators, tongue depressors, medicine cup to mix in medications

- Nasal cavity and nasopharynx anesthesia begin with using vasoconstricting agents to help minimize nasal bleeding and edema.
- This can be achieved by using *topical vasoconstrictors* such as *oxymetazoline*, phenylephrine, or cocaine (Table 7.2).
- Best to anesthetize both nares in case one is more patent than the other.
  - *Cocaine* is an ester that acts as a local anesthetic as well as a vasoconstrictor and comes in 1–4% solution or paste.
    Cocaine can be applied with soaked cotton-tip applicators along the floor of the nasal cavity and interior turbinate, advancing 1 cm at a time after allowing 30–60 seconds of time to absorb locally.

TABLE 7.2 Information on vasoconstrictors [20]

Vasoconstrictor	Preparation	Time of onset	Duration	Side effects	Max dose
Oxymetazoline	0.05% solution	10 min	12 h	Dry nose, nasal mucosa irritation	2–3 sprays/ nare
Phenylephrine	0.25–1% solution	2 min	2.4–4 h	Burning sensation, nasal discharge	2–3 sprays/ nare
Cocaine	4% solution	1 min	30 min	Headache, epistaxis, hypertension, tachycardia, angina, thyrotoxicosis	3 mg/kg

The cotton-tip can be removed and re-soaked in cocaine until it has touched the posterior wall of the nasal cavity, usually around 10 cm deep.

As the nasal tract opens, a second soaked cotton-tip applicator can be advanced just behind to the first to allow for formation of a wider tract.

Cocaine sympathomimetic effects include hypertension, angina, and thyrotoxicosis; caution should be taken for patients who are on monoamine oxidase inhibitor medications.

– *Lidocaine gel* (2–4%) *with phenylephrine* (0.25– 1%) in a 3:1 ratio or lidocaine gel with 2–3 mL of oxymetazoline mixture in a 3:1 ratio.

Mixture can be placed with the same cotton tip applicators and left in place for 10 minutes to allow for anesthesia and vasoconstriction.

An atomizer can also be used along the nasal tract followed by an increasing diameter of nasal trumpets coated with lidocaine jelly [10, 15, 19].

– Other options for anesthesia include the following:
One spray of the 10% lidocaine into the nasal mucosa or using the lidocaine-post-nasal-dripping (LPND) method.

In LPND, 10 mL of 2% lidocaine is drawn up into a 10 mL syringe that is connected to a two-inch #16-gauge catheter.

While the most patent nare is being vasoconstricted, the catheter is inserted into the nare that is not being vasoconstricted and allowed to drip until it elicits a cough reflex.

The cough reflex is thought to help spread the local anesthetic around the supraglottic area. If no cough reflex is elicited, the total 10 mL of anesthesia is dripped [21].

Oral Cavity and Oropharynx

Lidocaine is an amide with good mucosal absorption; max dose of lidocaine does not exceed 5 mg/kg

- Nebulizing local anesthetic, such as lidocaine, to the entire airway can minimize fluctuations in blood pressure and heart rate that comes from the gag reflex.
- 5 mL of 4% lidocaine can be nebulized with oxygen at flow <6 L/min so that larger droplets greater than 60 microns in size can precipitate out into the proximal airway.
- Higher flow of oxygen will create smaller droplets less than 30 microns in size that can travel further distally into bronchial tree and increase the rate of systemic absorption.
- 15–20 minutes are needed for inhaled topical anesthesia to be effective while the patient is sitting upright during nebulization.
- Nebulized lidocaine can have variable efficacy.
- Topical application of doses higher than 5 mg/kg may cause symptoms of toxicity including perioral numbness, seizures, respiratory failure, hypertension, ventricular arrhythmias with progressive hypotension [15, 22, 23].
- Other methods of oropharyngeal anesthesia include the following (Table 7.3):

TABLE 7.3 Information on topical anesthetics [20]

Anesthetic	Preparation	Concentration	Time of onset	Duration	Use	Max dose
Lidocaine	2% solution	20 mg/mL	3–5 min	15–30 min	Topical to oropharynx	5 mg/kg
	4% solution	40 mg/mL			Nebulization, topical to oropharynx	
	4% viscous gel	40 mg/mL			Lubricant to nasopharynx	
	5% ointment	50 mg/gm of ointment			Topical to oropharynx	
	10% spray	10 mg/dose			Topical application	
Cocaine	4% solution	40 mg/mL	1 min	30 min	Nasal vasoconstriction and anesthesia	3 mg/kg

- 10% lidocaine spray in the oral cavity as well as gargling viscous 2% lidocaine for 1–2 minutes and discard.
- Afterwards, 5% lidocaine ointment can be placed at the base of the tongue and allowed to melt prior to swallowing.

  Ointment is preferred over jelly as the ointment decreases in viscosity as it melts, allowing for a wider spread of anesthesia to the posterior and inferior pharynx and supraglottic area.

- In the "spray-as-you-go" method, the working channel of the fiberoptic scope can be used to instill lidocaine and anesthetize the supraglottic structure and vocal cords under direct visualization.
- This can also be done as a direct laryngoscope is advanced with the use of a malleable disposable atomizer wand such as MADgic® device.
- Lidocaine can be atomized or sprayed with 0.2–1 mL of 2% lidocaine, allowing 30 seconds for absorption and effect before advancing further into the airway [15, 17].

Benzocaine can also be used however it is currently not FDA-approved to use for anesthesia of mucous membranes as it holds the risk of benzocaine overdose and methemoglobinemia, causing it to fall out of favor for use [24].

Larynx Above and Below the Vocal Cords

- Anesthesia above and below the larynx can be obtained with the nebulized method as well as the "spray-as-you-go" method.
- Instilling lidocaine below and above the vocal cords will elicit a cough and this will help spread the anesthetic throughout the airway [10, 15, 19].
- Injections of *local anesthetics* to perform nerve blocks of the superior laryngeal nerve or performing trans-cricoid installation of lidocaine to anesthetize above and below the vocal cords are not ideal in an emergent setting [15]. Therefore, nerve blocks will not be covered in this chapter.

Step 3: Sedation and Analgesia

- If appropriate topical analgesia is performed, patients may require little-to-no sedation.
- However, despite effective anesthesia, there are pressure sensors at the base of the tongue that upon manipulation may illicit a gag reflex, laryngeal spasms, and cough, potentially exacerbating an already anxious patient.
- Medications selected should have a minimal effect on hemodynamics, airway tone, and respiratory effort (Table 7.4).
- Sedatives should also have rapid onset and be short acting.
- Sub-dissociative doses of *ketamine* can also be given in a slow bolus of 0.3–0.5 mg/kg doses over 5 minutes to help with discomfort, pain, and anxiety without suppressing respiratory drive.

TABLE 7.4 Information on sedatives [20]

Sedative	Use	Dose	Time of onset	Duration	Side effects
Ketamine	Sub-dissociative analgesic	IV: 0.3–0.5 mg/kg	IV: 30 sec IM: 3–4 min	IV: 5–10 min	Emergence psychosis, Hypertension, tachycardia
	Procedural	IV: 1–2 mg/kg IM: 4 mg/kg	IV: 30 sec IM: 3–4 min	IV: 5–10 min IM: 12–25 min	Emergence psychosis, Hypertension, tachycardia
Midazolam	Anxiolytic, Amnesia, sedation	IV: 0.5–2 mg	IV: 3–5 min	IV: 2 h	Respiratory depression
Fentanyl	Analgesic, sedation	IV: 1–2 mcg/kg	IV: 3–5 m min IM: 10–15 min	IV/IM: 30–45 min	Respiratory depression, bronchospasm, hypotension

- *Benzodiazepines* are often used as anxiolytics as well as for their antiemetic properties.
  - *Midazolam* is an ideal agent because it has a rapid onset, short half-life, and offers sedation and anterograde amnesia. Begin by giving 0.25 mg intravenous (IV) aliquots, with effects being seen in about 3 minutes.
- For pain and antitussive properties, opiates such as *fentanyl* are ideal as it is rapid-acting with short duration. Limit dosing to 50 mcg IV aliquots.
- Morphine takes longer for onset of action and can have effect on hemodynamics including hypotension and bronchospasm.
- Using both benzodiazepine and opiates together will have a synergistic effect, and when combined are effectively considered procedural sedation.

Mono therapy for awake intubation with or without the addition of topical anesthesia.

- Options include ketamine-only breathing intubation (KOBI), otherwise known as ketamine-assisted intubation, ketamine-facilitated intubation, ketamine-only intubation, ketamine-supported intubation, and dissociated awake intubation.

- A dissociative-dose of ketamine at 1–2 mg/kg IV or 4–6 mg/kg intramuscularly (IM), dosed at the ideal body weight, allows the patient to become amnestic while maintaining airway reflexes, respiration, and blood pressure.
- If glottic view is adequate and airway reflexes or vocal cord movement prevents successful tube placement, having readily available a fast-acting paralytic such as rocuronium or succinylcholine can aid with placement [9, 10].

Ketamine can be used as monotherapy, however any intubating technique used may lead to muscle rigidity, vomiting, laryngospasm or apnea.

What Equipment Do You Need?

- Awake intubation is usually performed with a flexible fiberoptic scope; however, this may not be feasible in many emergency departments due to both lack of emergent access and familiarity.
- Flexible fiberoptic scope assisted intubation can be performed via the nasal or oral route.
- To aid in the insertion of the fiberscope through the airway passage, a rigid hollow conduit must be utilized.
  - Nasal trumpet for the nasotracheal approach.
  - Williams airway for orotracheal approach.
- Additionally, a defogger can be applied to the tip of the fiberoptic scope prior to the procedure, as well as immersing the tip in warm saline or allow oxygen to flow though the suction port to serve as a defogging mechanism and increase fraction of inspired oxygen.
- Rigid laryngoscopes, which include both direct laryngoscopy (DL) and video laryngoscopy (VL), can also be utilized (Fig. 7.2).

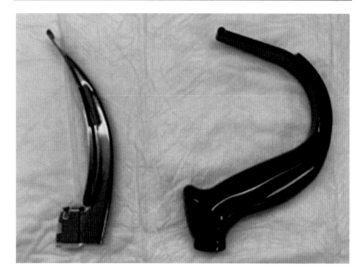

FIG. 7.2 Rigid laryngoscope examples. On the left is a Macintosh blade size #4, on the right is a hyperangulated Glidescope Spectrum Directview MAC S4

- These instruments can be very stimulating to the upper airways and require very good patient preparation with adequate anesthesia.
- Additionally, this approach can be very challenging in patients with limited ability to open the mouth, have space occupying lesions in the oral cavity or pharynx, or have limited cervical range of motion.
- Video laryngoscopes with their hyper-angulated blade and fixed wide view of the airway can aid in creating space within an airway allowing for adequate aspiration of secretions and blood under direct vision, aid in administration of atomized local anesthetics to glottis and trachea under direct view, and aid in visualizing placement of tracheal tube throughout the intubation process.
  - This is all done while minimizing airway trauma and reducing risk of impingement of the tube at the arytenoids [25].

Supraglottic Device

- In the unfortunate situation where an awake intubation fails, the airway collapses during the procedure, and the patient cannot be ventilated with a facemask, laryngeal mask airway (LMA) is a good backup.
- LMA is a type of supraglottic device which is a combination of an oropharyngeal airway and an ETT.
- Blindly, the LMA is advanced until resistance is felt; this is when the tip of the mask is assumed to be up against the esophagus.
- The inflatable rim is then inflated to provide a seal around the larynx.
- The tube of the LMA can be connected to a ventilator circuit and the opening in the center of the mask should allow for ventilation.
- Limitations for this airway include poor seal from inflatable rim, risk of aspiration, and patient must have ability to open mouth widely to application.
- LMA can be a temporizing measure until a more definitive airway can be obtained or planned for accordingly [19].

Failed Awake Intubation

- Common reasons for failure include the following:
  - Inadequate oropharyngeal or laryngeal anesthesia
  - Excessive secretions or blood
  - Difficult anatomy
  - Lack of patient cooperation
  - Over-sedation
  - Operator inexperience
- Above all, the biggest reason for failure of any endotracheal intubation is *failure to anticipate failure with no back-up plans*.
- It is vital to always devise a series of back-up plans so as to swiftly change approaches in case of difficulty.

- In the case of inadequate local anesthesia, before additional anesthetic agent is administered, make sure to calculate the total dose of local anesthesia *prior* to beginning the procedure to avoid toxicity.
- Although rare during an awake intubation, a patient may develop symptomatic complete airway obstruction that may lead to a "can't intubated, can't ventilate," situation with both bag-valve mask and LMA.
- Prior to awake intubation, always prepare by having sedatives and paralytics at bedside for potential induction for attempted airway intubation and, if available, assign another practitioner with a double setup to perform an emergency cricothyrotomy.

Bibliography

1. Soyuncu S, Eken C, Cete Y, Bektas F, Akcimen M. Determination of difficult intubation in the ED. Am J Emerg Med. 2009;27(8):905–10. https://doi.org/10.1016/j.ajem.2008.07.003. PubMed [citation] PMID: 19857405
2. Bair AE, Caravelli R, Tyler K, Laurin EG. Feasibility of the preoperative Mallampati airway assessment in emergency department patients. J Emerg Med. 2010;38(5):677–80. https://doi.org/10.1016/j.jemermed.2008.12.019. Epub 2009 Mar 17. PubMed [citation] PMID: 19297115
3. Levitan RM, Everett WW, Ochroch EA. Limitations of difficult airway prediction in patients intubated in the emergency department. Ann Emerg Med. 2004;44(4):307–13. PubMed [citation] PMID: 15459613
4. Law JA, Morris IR, Brousseau PA, de la Ronde S, Milne AD. The incidence, success rate, and complications of awake tracheal intubation in 1,554 patients over 12 years: an historical cohort study. Can J Anaesth. 2015;62(7):736–44. https://doi.org/10.1007/s12630-015-0387-y. Epub 2015 Apr 24. PubMed [citation] PMID: 25907462
5. Sakles JC, Douglas MJK, Hypes CD, Patanwala AE, Mosier JM. Management of patients with predicted difficult airways in an Academic Emergency Department. J Emerg Med. 2017;53(2):163–71. https://doi.org/10.1016/j.jemermed.2017.04.003. Epub 2017 Jun 9. PubMed [citation] PMID: 28606617

6. Allan AG. Reluctance of anaesthetists to perform awake intubation. Anaesthesia. 2004r;59(4):413. No abstract available. PubMed [citation] PMID: 15023129.

7. Brown CA 3rd, Bair AE, Pallin DJ, Walls RM, NEAR III Investigators. Techniques, success, and adverse events of emergency department adult intubations. Ann Emerg Med. 2015;65(4):363–370.e1. https://doi.org/10.1016/j.annemergmed.2014.10.036. Epub 2014 Dec 20. Erratum in: Ann Emerg Med. 2017 May;69(5):540. PubMed [citation] PMID: 25533140

8. Apfelbaum JL, Hagberg CA, Caplan RA, Blitt CD, Connis RT, Nickinovich DG, Hagberg CA, Caplan RA, Benumof JL, Berry FA, Blitt CD, Bode RH, Cheney FW, Connis RT, Guidry OF, Nickinovich DG, Ovassapian A, American Society of Anesthesiologists Task Force on Management of the Difficult Airway. Practice guidelines for management of the difficult airway: an updated report by the American Society of Anesthesiologists Task Force on Management of the Difficult Airway. Anesthesiology. 2013;118(2):251–70. https://doi.org/10.1097/ALN.0b013e31827773b2. No abstract available. PubMed [citation] PMID: 23364566

9. Merelman AH, Perlmutter MC, Strayer RJ. Alternatives to rapid sequence intubation: contemporary airway management with ketamine. West J Emerg Med. 2019;20(3):466–71. https://doi.org/10.5811/westjem.2019.4.42753. Epub 2019 Apr 26. Review. PubMed [citation] PMID: 31123547, PMCID: PMC6526883

10. Tonna JE, DeBlieux PM. Awake laryngoscopy in the emergency department. J Emerg Med. 2017;52(3):324–31. https://doi.org/10.1016/j.jemermed.2016.11.013. Epub 2016 Dec 12. PubMed [citation] PMID: 27979641

11. Abdelmalak B, Makary L, Hoban J, Doyle DJ. Dexmedetomidine as sole sedative for awake intubation in management of the critical airway. J Clin Anesth. 2007;19(5):370–3. PubMed [citation] PMID: 17869990

12. Joseph TT, Gal JS, DeMaria S Jr, Lin HM, Levine AI, Hyman JB. A retrospective study of success, failure, and time needed to perform awake intubation. Anesthesiology. 2016;125(1):105–14. https://doi.org/10.1097/ALN.0000000000001140. PubMed [citation] PMID: 27111535

13. Mosier JM, Hypes CD, Sakles JC. Understanding preoxygenation and apneic oxygenation during intubation in the critically ill. Intensive Care Med. 2017;43(2):226–8. https://doi.org/10.1007/s00134-016-4426-0. Epub 2016 Jun 24. No abstract available. PubMed [citation] PMID: 27342820

14. Law JA, Broemling N, Cooper RM, Drolet P, Duggan LV, Griesdale DE, Hung OR, Jones PM, Kovacs G, Massey S, Morris IR, Mullen T, Murphy MF, Preston R, Naik VN, Scott J, Stacey S, Turkstra TP, Wong DT, Canadian Airway Focus Group. The difficult airway with recommendations for management--part 2--the anticipated difficult airway. Can J Anaesth. 2013;60(11):1119–38. https://doi.org/10.1007/s12630-013-0020-x. Epub 2013 Oct 17. PubMed [citation] PMID: 24132408, PMCID: PMC3825645

15. Walsh ME, Shorten GD. Preparing to perform an awake fiberoptic intubation. Yale J Biol Med. 1998;71(6):537–49. Review. PubMed [citation] PMID: 10604785, PMCID: PMC2578951

16. Ahmed A, Azim A. Difficult tracheal intubation in critically ill. J Intensive Care. 2018;6:49. https://doi.org/10.1186/s40560-018-0318-4. eCollection 2018. Review. PubMed [citation] PMID: 30123510, PMCID: PMC6090786

17. Doyle DJ. Airway anesthesia: theory and practice. Anesthesiol Clin. 2015;33(2):291–304. https://doi.org/10.1016/j.anclin.2015.02.013. Review. PubMed [citation]. PMID: 25999003

18. Simmons ST, Schleich AR. Airway regional anesthesia for awake fiberoptic intubation. Reg Anesth Pain Med. 2002;27(2):180–92. Review. No abstract available. PubMed [citation] PMID: 11915066

19. Benumof JL. Management of the difficult adult airway. With special emphasis on awake tracheal intubation. Anesthesiology. 1991;75(6):1087–110. Review. Erratum in: Anesthesiology 1993 Jan;78(1):224. PubMed [citation] PMID: 1824555

20. Wolters Kluwer Clinical Drug Information, Inc. (Lexi-drugs). Wolters Kluwer clinical drug Information, Inc; September 18, 2019.

21. Sukhupragarn W, Leurcharusmee P. Lidocaine post-nasal dripping (LPND): an easy way for awake nasal intubation. J Clin Anesth. 2018;44:105–6. https://doi.org/10.1016/j.jclinane.2017.11.022. Epub 2017 Nov 23. No abstract available. PubMed [citation] PMID: 29175751

22. Kumar M, Chawla R, Goyal M. Topical anesthesia. J Anaesthesiol Clin Pharmacol. 2015;31(4):450–6. https://doi.org/10.4103/0970-9185.169049. Review. PubMed [citation] PMID: 26702198, PMCID: PMC4676230

23. Sutherland AD, Williams RT. Cardiovascular responses and lidocaine absorption in fiberoptic-assisted awake intubation. Anesth Analg. 1986;65(4):389–91. PubMed [citation] PMID: 3954113

24. United States, Federal Drug Administration. Safety Information on Benzocaine-Containing Products. Federal Register, 15 June 2018, www.fda.gov/drugs/postmarket-drug-safety-information-patients-and-providers/safety-information-benzocaine-containing-products. Accessed 19 Sept. 2019.

25. Fitzgerald E, Hodzovic I, Smith AF. 'From darkness into light': time to make awake intubation with videolaryngoscopy the primary technique for an anticipated difficult airway? Anaesthesia. 2015;70(4):387–92. https://doi.org/10.1111/anae.13042. No abstract available. PubMed [citation] PMID: 25764402

Chapter 8
Now the Tube Is In: Post-Intubation Sedation

Colleen Barthol

Key Points
- Intubation and mechanical ventilation can induce emotional and physical distress.
- Patients must not endure chemical paralysis without sedation in the immediate post-intubation period.
- Evidence-based guidelines for evaluation of pain and agitation can help guide therapy.
- Be aware of possible side effects and toxicities of your sedative agents.

Pain Assessment and Use of Analgesics

- The Society of Critical Care Medicine 2018 guidelines for Pain, Agitation, Delirium, Immobility and Sleep Disruption (PADIS) recommend using an assessment-driven, protocol-based, stepwise approach for pain and sedation management in critically ill adults [4]

C. Barthol (✉)
Department of Pharmacotherapy & Pharmacy Services, University Health System, San Antonio, TX, USA
e-mail: Colleen.Barthol@uhs-sa.com

© Springer Nature Switzerland AG 2021
R. Garvin (ed.), *Intubating the Critically Ill Patient*,
https://doi.org/10.1007/978-3-030-56813-9_8

TABLE 8.1 Comparison of analgesics [2, 5]

Analgesic	Onset	Dosing	Precautions	Pearls
Fentanyl	1–2 min	0.35–0.5 mcg/kg IV q30–60 min or 0.7–10 mcg/kg/hr	Highly lipophilic Chest wall rigidity with high doses or rapid IV bolus	Most hemodynamically neutral
Hydromorphone	5–15 min	0.2–0.6 mg IV q1-2hr or 0.5–3 mg/hr	Accumulation with hepatic/ renal impairment	Approximately 5× potency of morphine
Morphine	5–10 min	2–4 mg IV q1-2hr or 2–30 mg/hr	Histamine release; hypotension Active metabolites M6G and M3G[a] can accumulate in renal failure	Frequently used to relieve chest pain
Remifentanil	1–3 min	1.5 mcg/kg IV → 0.5–15 mcg/kg/hr	Ultra-short acting	Rapid metabolism via blood and tissue esterases
Ketamine [6]	30 sec	0.2–0.8 mg/kg IV → 1–20 mcg/kg/min	Hypertension and tachycardia Emergence reactions	Causes bronchodilation

[a]*M6G* morphine-6-glucuronide, *M3G* morphine-3-glucuronide

- Pain assessment should be performed using either the Behavioral Pain Scale (BPS) or Critical Care Pain Observation Tool (CPOT), as these demonstrate the greatest validity and reliability for monitoring pain in critically ill patients [4]
- Pain scales for ICU patients take into account a patient's inability to verbalize their discomfort.
- Opioids, such as fentanyl, remain the mainstay for pain management.
- Incorporating multimodal pharmacotherapy including use of acetaminophen, ketamine, lidocaine, neuropathic agents and nonsteroidal anti-inflammatory agents is recommended (Table 8.1) [4]

Sedation Assessment and Use of Sedatives

- Sedatives are frequently administered to relieve anxiety, reduce stress of mechanical ventilation and prevent agitation-related harm [4]
- Sedation assessment should be performed with a validated tool such as Richmond Agitation Sedation Scale (RASS) or Sedation Agitation Scale (SAS) [4]
- Sedation assessments should occur at least hourly in ICU patients or more frequently as needed.
- The goal for the majority of ICU patient is a RASS score between 0 to 1; between alert and calm and opening eyes to voice.
- Groth et al. reported delays in post-RSI sedation following administration of non-depolarizing neuromuscular blocking agents (NDNMBA) [3]
  - Approximately 80% did not receive adequate sedation post-NDNMBA use taking into consideration the duration of action of the induction agent.
  - Nearly 30% did not receive any sedation within the first 120 min.
- However, not all mechanically ventilated patients require sedatives; each patient should be evaluated individually.
- Non-benzodiazepine sedatives (i.e., propofol or dexmedetomidine) are preferred in critically ill, mechanically ventilated patients because of improved short-term outcomes such as ICU length of stay, duration of mechanical ventilation, and delirium [2]
- Short-acting agents are ideal in the ED/ICU setting due to the ability to quickly evaluate neurologic status.
- Consider the hemodynamic profile when choosing medications.
  - Ketamine can be advantageous for sedation and analgesia in patients with persistent hypotension due to its sympathomimetic effects.
  - Propofol can be helpful for agitated and hypertensive patients due to its cardiodepressant effects (Table 8.2).

TABLE 8.2 Comparison of sedatives [2, 5]

Sedative	Onset	Dosing	Precautions	Pearls
Dexmedetomidine	5–10 min	0.2–1.5 mcg/kg/hr	Hypotension and bradycardia	Minimal respiratory depression Only sedative approved for administration in non-intubated ICU patients
Ketamine	30 sec	0.5–4 mg/kg/hr [8]	Hypertension and tachycardia Emergence reactions Acute myocardial infarction or decompensated heart failure	Analgesic, sedative, dissociative, anticonvulsant properties
Lorazepam	2–3 min	0.02–0.04 mg/kg IV loading dose 0.01–0.1 mg/kg/hr	High dose and prolonged infusions can lead to propylene glycol toxicity	Contains propylene glycol; Preferred benzo for elderly and cirrhotics
Midazolam	2–5 min	0.01–0.05 mg/kg IV loading dose 0.02–0.1 mg/kg/hr	Respiratory depression and hypotension; active metabolite 1-hydroxy-midazolam can accumulate in renal failure	Does not contain propylene glycol
Propofol	1–2 min	5–50 mcg/kg/min	Hypotension and bradycardia Lipid base (1 kcal/mL) can lead to hypertriglyceridemia Propofol infusion syndrome	Can lower intracranial pressure Can cause green discoloration of urine, a rare and benign side effect

- *Do not use your sedatives to manage blood pressure*; instead, make sure that pain or agitation is not causing the blood pressure increase.

Know What to Watch For

- Propylene glycol (PG) toxicity [7]
  - PG is a solvent for intravenous, oral, and topical pharmaceutical preparations.
  - PG is found in sedatives like intravenous diazepam, lorazepam and pentobarbital.
  - Toxicity can occur with accumulation of PG during high doses or prolonged infusions.
  - Signs/symptoms of PG toxicity include anion gap hyperosmolar metabolic acidosis, acute kidney injury, cardiac arrhythmias, and seizures.
  - Management includes stopping the offending medication and hemodialysis in severe cases.
- Propofol-related infusion syndrome (PRIS) [1]
  - Rare, but life-threatening complication presenting as metabolic acidosis, rhabdomyolysis, dysrhythmias, and progression of cardiac/renal failure.
  - More common with higher doses and prolonged infusions.
  - Management requires immediate discontinuation of propofol and supportive care.

References

1. Wood S, Winters ME. Care of the intubated emergency department patient. J Em Med. 2011;40(4):419–27.
2. Barr J, Fraser GL, Puntillo K, et al. Clinical practice guidelines for the management of pain, agitation, and delirium in adult patients in the intensive care unit. Crit Care Med. 2013;41:263–306.
3. Groth CM, Acquisto NM, Khadem T. Current practices and safety of medication use during rapid sequence intubation. J Crit Care. 2018;45:65–70.
4. Devlin JW, Skrobik Y, Gelinas C, et al. Clinical practice guidelines for the prevention and management of pain, agitation/sedation, delirium, immobility, and sleep disruption in adult patients in the ICU. Crit Care Med. 2018;46(9):1–49.

5. Lexicomp Online, Hudson, Ohio: Wolters Kluwer clinical drug information, Inc; 2019; October 12, 2019.
6. Erstad BL, Patanwala AE. Ketamine for Analgosedation in critically ill patients. J Crit Care. 2016;35:145–9.
7. Arroliga A, Shehab N, McCarthy K, Gonzales J. Relationship of continuous infusion lorazepam to serum propylene glycol concentration in critically ill adults. Crit Care Med. 2004;32(8):1709–14.
8. Umunna BP, Tekwani K, Kulstad E. Ketamine for continuous sedation of mechanically ventilated patients. J Emerg Trauma Shock. 2015;8(1):11–5.

Chapter 9
The Cardiac Patient

Kari Gorder and Jordan B. Bonomo

> **Key Points**
> - Patients with acute myocardial infarctions, cardiogenic shock, right ventricular failure, and acute valvular disorders present an added challenge to the already complex physiology of peri-intubation hemodynamics.
> - The addition of positive-pressure ventilation and positive-end expiratory pressure can decrease right-sided venous return and contribute to decreases in cardiac output in patients who are hypovolemic or particularly pressure-sensitive, and must be done with caution.
> - Anticipation and management of this physiology require a pro-active strategy which may include volume expansion, vasopressor or inotrope administration, or the addition of invasive monitoring devices.

K. Gorder (✉)
The Christ Hospital and Lindner Institute for Research and Education, Cincinnati, OH, USA
e-mail: kari.gorder@thechristhospital.com

J. B. Bonomo
Department of Emergency Medicine, University of Cincinnati College of Medicine, Cincinnati, OH, USA
e-mail: bonomojb@ucmail.uc.edu

© Springer Nature Switzerland AG 2021
R. Garvin (ed.), *Intubating the Critically Ill Patient*,
https://doi.org/10.1007/978-3-030-56813-9_9

- Calculating the shock index may allow for anticipation of which patient will develop post-intubation hypotension.
- Thoughtful pharmacologic choices for induction medications can mitigate some of the consequences of intubation in this complex patient population.

General Principles

- Due to the complex interplay between cardiac output, oxygen-carrying capacity, and cardiopulmonary reserve, hypoxemia and hypercarbia are often poorly tolerated in patients with underlying cardiac disease.
- Even brief periods of inadequate oxygenation or ventilation can precipitate significant or irreversible hemodynamic collapse.
- Early anticipation of the need for advanced airway management in cardiac patients can facilitate the adequate preparation, optimization of hemodynamics, and acquisition of resources that these patients often require.
- Delayed sequence intubation [1], which temporally separates the sedative and paralytic agents, allows for adequate preoxygenation in the interim via multiple methods and should be considered for unstable cardiac patients who cannot be safely preoxygenated using standard RSI techniques.
- The method of laryngoscopy with which the operator is most familiar should be used, with special attention to how the patient's underlying cardiac physiology may influence hemodynamics.

Management of Peri-Intubation Hemodynamics

- Myocardial Oxygen Demand
  - For patients with underlying cardiovascular disease, myocardial oxygen demand is an important physiologic

parameter that can become perturbed in the peri-intubation period.

- Hypertension and tachycardia are common during the initial physical manipulation of the airway [2], via neuroendocrine pathways modulated by the sympathetic nervous system.
- The primary components of myocardial oxygen demand are *myocardial wall tension* and *heart rate.*
- Tachycardia both directly increases myocardial oxygen consumption and reduces diastolic filling time and relaxation, increasing myocardial wall stress and myocardial ischemia.
- Consequently, peri-intubation tachycardia can be particularly stressful for the patient with underlying active cardiovascular disease.
- Blunting of the hypertensive and tachycardic responses to airway manipulation should be attempted via appropriate induction agents and analgosedation in patients at high risk for myocardial ischemia, such as in patients with active acute coronary syndrome (ACS).
- For patients with aortic disease such as aortic dissection or aneurysmal dilation of the aorta, every effort should be made to minimize abrupt increases in blood pressure or heart rate, as this can increase transmural wall tension and have devastating consequences.

- Effects on Systemic Venous Return
  - The effect of the transition from negative-pressure, spontaneous ventilation to positive-pressure, mechanical ventilation cannot be understated in the patient with cardiovascular disease.
  - Positive pressure increases intrathoracic pressure, which can disrupt the low venous pressure required by the right heart for adequate venous return.
  - When blood return to the right side of the heart is diminished, blood flow through the pulmonary vasculature is altered, leading to decreased left ventricular preload.
    - While compensatory tachycardia and increases in systemic tone may occur, many critically ill cardiac

patients do not possess the catecholaminergic reserve to adequately compensate for this decreased volume, and subsequently cardiac output and mean arterial pressure fall [3].

- Sedatives and paralytics may cause vasodilation or adrenergic blunting, exacerbating this response. This effect may also be exacerbated in patients with primary right ventricular dysfunction, as discussed below.
- Conversely, positive pressure can be at times therapeutic for the critically ill cardiac patient, depending on the pre-intubation interplay between the patient's preload and afterload status.
- The increased intrathoracic pressure of positive-pressure ventilation decreases the left ventricular transmural gradient and subsequently decreases left ventricular afterload.
- This decrease in afterload may directly increase cardiac output in cardiogenic shock patients who are primarily afterload sensitive.
- There is some evidence that, by decreasing left ventricular afterload, positive-pressure ventilation may also decrease left ventricular wall tension and myocardial oxygen demand. [4–6]
- Whether this actually translates to improved cardiac output is still a matter of debate [7].
- In cases of cardiogenic shock, care must be taken to anticipate and respond to the potential hemodynamic consequences of positive pressure ventilation.
- For some patients, positive-end expiratory pressure (PEEP)-mediated reduction in cardiac output may be volume-responsive [8], and the provider must be prepared to counteract peri-intubation hypotension with volume expansion.
- In other clinical scenarios, such as the hypervolemic heart failure patient, additional volume may exacerbate the underlying pathology; in these patients, administration of peri-intubation "push-dose" pres-

sors or the pre-intubation initiation of other vasoactive agents may improve an otherwise rocky hemodynamic course, as discussed below.

- Blunting of Adrenergic Response and Post-Intubation Hypotension
  - Unstable cardiac patients are in a state of adrenergic upregulation as a compensatory mechanism to maintain adequate cardiac output.
  - The sympatholysis that occurs with administration of a rapidly acting sedative or hypnotic, as is often done during RSI, is one of several well-known causes of post-intubation hypotension.
  - Between 25% and 46% of all patients in the ED or ICU undergoing RSI will experience post-intubation hypotension [9, 10], which is independently associated with increased morbidity and mortality.
  - The *shock index (SI),* calculated as a ratio of heart rate to systolic blood pressure, is an early predictor of shock in the setting of otherwise reassuring vital signs.
  - A normal shock index is 0.5–0.7, and an elevated SI is associated with the likelihood of post-intubation hypotension [11].
  - This value, among other known predictors of post-intubation hypotension such as advanced age, known left ventricular dysfunction, and other comorbid disease, can help the clinician predict and prepare for post-intubation hypotension with pharmacologic management and support.

Pharmacologic Management

The pharmacologic management surrounding the intubation of patients in cardiogenic shock centers around providing a *hemodynamically neutral induction.* Dose reduction or avoidance of certain typical RSI agents may be necessary in this patient population.

Induction Agents

Etomidate

- A short-acting intravenous sedative agent, etomidate has relatively neutral effects on cardiac output and blood pressure, and has been shown in some observational studies to have minimal hemodynamic effects on shocked patients [12].
- It is typically given at a dose of 0.15–0.3 mg/kg IV.
- A recent study [13] investigating the pharmacology of RSI showed that only dose reduction of etomidate had a significant impact on decreasing the incidence of postintubation hypotension when compared to modulating the dose of other RSI sedation drugs.
- Etomidate is not thought to blunt the stimulating effects of upper airway manipulation, which, as discussed previously, may lead to hypertension or tachycardia that can increase myocardial oxygen demand in select cardiac patients.
- Addition of pretreatment medications such as opioids may be considered for patients for whom this is a primary hemodynamic concern.

Propofol

- Has generally fallen out of favor as a sedative agent in RSI for the shocked patient due to its propensity to induce hypotension.
- Typically dosed at 1–2 mg/kg for induction, some authors suggest a significant dose reduction to 0.1–0.4 mg/kg in patients with hemodynamic instability [14].
- However, with a longer duration to effect than other sedative agents, propofol is unlikely to be the agent of choice for the emergent airway in the cardiac patient.

Ketamine

- A dissociative anesthetic that has a relatively short time to onset (typically less than 1 minute).

- At a dose of 1–2 mg/kg for induction, ketamine is relatively unique in its ability to preserve respiratory drive while precipitating sedation.
- For the cardiac patient, this can help avoid the deleterious consequences of hypoxemia on the heart.
- Ketamine also causes sympathetic stimulation, typically leading to an elevated blood pressure and heart rate, an attractive physiologic parameter in the shocked cardiac patient.
- However, some studies have shown that in the catecholamine-deplete patient, ketamine can cause peri-intubation hypotension and in fact has the ability to be a direct myocardial depressant [15].
- This may be predicted in patients with elevated shock indices, as discussed above [16].
- Depending on the etiology for the patient's cardiac collapse, ketamine may not be the drug of choice for induction.

Other Agents

Benzodiazepines

- Midazolam is likely the most commonly used benzodiazepine due to its shorter duration to action.
- It is classically dosed at 0.1–0.3 mg/kg for induction, although it has been found to be frequently under-dosed in this setting, potentially due to providers' unfamiliarity with induction dosing [17].
- While hypotension is commonly seen at intubating doses, some providers continue to use benzodiazepines for the intubation of critically ill patients with success [18].
- Some authors recommend using small doses of intravenous benzodiazepines over a longer period of time in the peri-intubation period of a shocked patient, should the clinical scenario allow it [19].
- As benzodiazepines offer no analgesic effect, an opioid such as fentanyl is frequently co-administered if no other pharmacologic agents are to be used in RSI. This strategy may afford the provider time for additional preoxygenation in a delayed sequence intubation fashion.

Neuromuscular Blocking Agents

- Studies have shown improved post-intubation hemodynamics in all patients who received neuromuscular blocking agents compared to those that did not [20].
- At least one study has shown that the incidence of post-intubation hypotension was higher in patients receiving succinylcholine over non-depolarizing drugs, such as rocuronium [21].
- In general, the use of neuromuscular blockade for RSI increases the rate of first-pass success and reduced complications in the intubation of the critically ill cardiac patient.

Fentanyl

- Often discussed as an adjunctive agent during RSI to blunt pain-mediated responses during the process of intubation, which can be of critical importance for some cardiac patients, such as the individual with an acute aortic dissection.
- The dose of fentanyl required to prevent peri-intubation hypertension and tachycardia, however, is described in the literature as anywhere from 2 mcg/kg to 15 mcg/kg [22, 23], with only higher doses observing adequate suppression of undesired hemodynamic response to intubation.
- As per some studies, intravenous fentanyl requires *over 5 minutes* from administration to achieve effect-site equilibrium, and thus cannot be given as a rapid push with standard induction agents [24].
- Although less frequently experienced than with other opioids, hypotension may be seen with fentanyl administration as well.

Topical Lidocaine

- Described in the literature as a method by which hemodynamic responses to physical stimulation of the airway may be blunted [25].

- However, the hemodynamic significance of this is unclear, and instillation of topical lidocaine can also cause bradycardia and other unwanted hemodynamic effects [26].
- As such, topical anesthetics *are not* recommended in the intubation of the cardiac patient outside of adjunctive use in delayed sequence intubation [27].

Inotropes and Vasopressors

- Bolus administration of vasopressors, frequently referred to as "push-dose pressors," is an increasingly common method of mitigating acute hypotension in the ED or ICU setting.
- Push-dose pressors have the ability to acutely stabilize a patient's hemodynamics while initiating continuous infusions of vasopressors or inotropes.
- While robust evidence surrounding the use of push-dose pressors in the shocked patient is lacking, retrospective studies have suggested their efficacy and safety in this setting [28], while highlighting the concern for dosing errors.
- The most commonly used bolus dose vasopressors in the critical care arena are *phenylephrine* and *epinephrine*, and, while easy to make at the bedside, are often stocked in pre-filled syringes in many EDs and ICUs.
  - *Phenylephrine*, an alpha agonist, has no direct inotropic effect but can lead to increased cardiac output precipitated by improved systemic venous return.
      With a time to onset of less than 1 minute, bolus doses of 50–200 mcg can be used both before and after intubation to maintain systemic pressures.
      Reflex bradycardia may occur with this agent.
  - *Epinephrine*, a mixed alpha and beta agonist, has some degree of inotropic support for the shocked cardiac patient. With an equally short time to onset as phenylephrine:
      Push doses of 5–20 mcg are usually adequate to support hemodynamics.
      Tachydysrhythmias are a common side effect of epinephrine use.

Specific Scenarios

Cardiogenic Shock: "Resuscitate Before you Intubate"

- Cardiogenic shock occurs in patients with low cardiac output states with evidence of end-organ dysfunction.
- Clinical criteria for the diagnosis of cardiogenic shock include hypotension, elevated lactate, altered mental status, and renal dysfunction.
- Cardiogenic shock remains a frequent and deadly consequence for the patient with acute myocardial infarction (AMI), with mortality rates exceeding 50% in some cases.
- While AMI remains the leading cause of cardiogenic shock, it is a multi-factorial condition with myriad etiologies and complex hemodynamics.
- Hemodynamic criteria include low cardiac indices (<1.8 l/min/m^2 for patients not on inotropic support, or <2.2 l/min/m^2 for those requiring inotropes), elevated pulmonary capillary wedge pressure (>15 mmHg), or a pulmonary artery pulsatility index (PAPi) of less than 1.0 [29].
- Consensus statements recommend a low threshold for initiating mechanical ventilation, acknowledging the high prevalence of respiratory failure in this patient population [30], and the significant effect that metabolic derangements can have on the shocked heart.
- Patients who are hypotensive preceding intubation have a significantly higher mortality rate than those who are hemodynamically stable [31].
- When preparing to intubate a hypotensive patient in cardiogenic shock, one should attempt to improve hemodynamics prior to intubation by means of volume, pressors, or inotropes.

Right Ventricular (RV) Failure

- The right ventricle (RV) is a low-pressure system and is exquisitely sensitive to changes in preload, afterload, and contractility.

- RV failure occurs when the struggling right ventricle is no longer able to generate sufficient pressure to maintain adequate blood flow through the pulmonary vasculature, ultimately decreasing left ventricular preload and thus cardiac output.
- This can be due to an acute condition such as right-sided myocardial infarction, massive pulmonary embolism (PE), or an acute-on-chronic process such as severe pulmonary hypertension.
- When the RV experiences increased afterload, this can precipitate a downward spiral of increased RV wall tension, decreased RV perfusion, and contractility.
- For the patient with acute RV failure or severe pulmonary hypertension, effects of PEEP can be magnified and are of significant clinical importance.
- Simply increasing lung volume via positive-pressure ventilation can increase pulmonary vascular resistance by directly compressing alveolar vessels [32].
- The complex interdependence between venous return, ventricular interdependence, and pulmonary pressures can be easily disrupted via the addition of PEEP, leading to increased RV afterload and decreased left ventricle (LV) function.
- Optimization of RV function prior to intubation is imperative, and may require intravascular volume expansion, aggressive correction of acid/base disorders, the addition of intravenous vasoactive agents, or the initiation of *inhaled pulmonary vasodilators*.
  - *Nitric oxide* and *epoprostenol* are two examples of inhaled agents that act as pulmonary vasodilators, thereby decreasing RV afterload.
  - Such agents can be initiated prior to or after intubation, and, although they may occasionally have unwanted systemic hemodynamic effects, are typically well tolerated [33].

Valvular Disease

- Patients with acute, severe valvular disorders may present in extremis and in need of expeditious resuscitation and management.
- Valvular emergencies include acute valvular regurgitation and, less often, stenosis.
- Precipitating etiologies may include endocarditis, ischemia, chordal rupture, post-surgical or post-procedural complications, prosthetic valve dysfunction, trauma, and genetic factors.
- These valvular disorders may tip the balance of already frail and complex hemodynamics toward profound cardiogenic or, in some instances, obstructive shock.
  - *Aortic and mitral valve regurgitation are preload dependent and afterload sensitive.*
    - In the most severe cases, patients may present with hypotension, pulmonary edema, and respiratory distress.
    - Hemodynamic goals surrounding intubation should focus on maintaining adequate preload while managing afterload and ensuring LV contractility.
    - Acute valvular regurgitation has less compensated ventricular function compared to acute-on-chronic disease, and thus less able to cope with acute ventricular overload.
    - The choice of induction agent should take into account the extent of myocardial depression.
    - Hemodynamic goals surrounding intubation should focus on adequate preload, which often requires the administration of fluid and maintenance of contractility, which may necessitate the initiation of a vasoactive medication such as norepinephrine or dobutamine.
    - For patients with post-intubation hypertension, short-acting vasodilators such as nitroglycerin, or hydralazine can be used to decrease afterload and promote forward flow [34].

- *Aortic and mitral stenosis may cause particular sensitivity to hypoxia or hypercarbia*, both of which can precipitate pulmonary vasoconstriction and worsen their disease process.
  - In its most severe form, left-sided valvular stenosis can lead to hypotension, pulmonary edema, RV dysfunction, and cardiovascular collapse.
  - Intubation should be done with special consideration to avoid tachycardia (in order to increase diastolic filling time of the left ventricle) and toward any actions that may increase pulmonary pressures, such as the use of alpha-adrenergic agents.
  - For patients with acute dysrhythmias in this setting, establishment of sinus rhythm prior to intubation may allow for improved diastolic filling [34].

Cardiac Arrest

- As our understanding of cardiac arrest treatment has progressed, organizations such as the American Heart Association have emphasized the prioritization of hands-only bystander cardiopulmonary resuscitation (CPR) and continuous chest compressions.
- The Advanced Cardiac Life Support (ACLS) guidelines now recommend that *chest compressions should not be stopped in order to place an advanced airway*, unless the patient cannot be bag-mask ventilated [35].
- Prehospital literature has highlighted that advanced airway management may be associated with worse neurologic outcomes [36], and recent studies have shown that even for in-hospital cardiac arrests, initiation of early tracheal intubation is associated with decreased survival to discharge [37].
- As such, for the patient in active cardiac arrest in the ED or ICU, quality bag-mask ventilation or the use of a supraglottic device may be sufficient for airway management until definitive return of spontaneous circulation has been achieved.

References

1. Weingart S, Trueger S, et al. Delayed sequence intubation: a prospective observational study. Ann Emerg Med. 2014;65:349–55.
2. Dorsey DP, Joffe AM. Physiologic and pathophysiologic responses to intubation. In: Hagberg CA, Artime CA, Aziz MF, editors. Hagberg and Benumof's Airway management. 4th ed. Elsevier: Philidelphia; PA. 2018.
3. Wiesen J, Ornstein M, et al. State of the evidence: mechanical ventilation with PEEP in patients with cardiogenic shock. Heart. 2013;99:1812–7.
4. Wiesen J, Ornstein M, et al. State of the evidence: mechanical ventilation with PEEP in patients with cardiogenic shock. Heart. 2013;99:1812–7.
5. Gomez H, Pinsky MR. Effect of mechanical ventilation on heart-lung interactions. In: Tobin M, editor. Principles and practice of mechanical ventilation. McGraw Hill: New York; 2013.
6. Grace MP, Greenbaum DM. Cardiac performance in response to PEEP in patients with cardiac dysfunction. Crit Care Med. 1982;10:358–60.
7. Fellahi JL, et al. Does positive end-expiratory pressure ventilation improve left ventricular function? A comparative study by transesophageal echocardiography in cardiac and noncardiac patients. Chest. 1998;114:556.
8. Gomez H, Pinsky MR. Effect of mechanical ventilation on heart-lung interactions. In: Tobin M, editor. Principles and practice of mechanical ventilation: McGraw Hill; 2013.
9. Heffener AC, et al. The frequency and significance of postintubation hypotension during emergency airway management. J Crit Care. 2012;27:417.e9–417.e13.
10. Green RS, et al. Postintubation hypotension in intensive care unit patients: a multicenter cohort study. J Crit Care. 2015;30:1055–60.
11. Heffener AC, et al. Predictors of the complications of postintubation hypotension during emergency airway management. J Crit Care. 2012;27:587–93.
12. Zed PJ, Abu-Laban RB, Harrison DW. Intubating conditions and hemodynamic effects of etomidate for rapid sequence intubation in the emergency department: an observational cohort study. Acad Emerg Med. 2006;13:378–83.
13. Kim JM, et al. Sedative dose and patient variable impacts on postintubation hypotension in emergency airway management. Am J Emerg Med. 2019;37:1248–53.

14. Manthous C. Avoiding circulatory complications during endotracheal intubation and initiation of positive pressure ventilation. J Emerg Med. 2010;38:633–1.
15. Sprung J, Schuetz S, et al. Effects of ketamine on the contractility of failing and nonfailing human heart muscles in vitro. Anesthesiology. 1998;88:1202–10.
16. Miller M, et al. Hemodynamic response after rapid sequence induction with ketamine in out of hospital patients at risk of shock as defined by the shock index. Ann Emerg Med. 2016;68:181.
17. Sagarin MJ, Barton ED, et al. Underdosing of midazolam in emergency endotracheal intubation. Ann Emerg Med. 2003;10:329–38.
18. Gherke L, et al. Diazepam or midazolam for orotracheal intubation in the ICU? Rev Assoc Med Bras. 2015;61:30–4.
19. Manthous C. Avoiding circulatory complications during endotracheal intubation and initiation of positive pressure ventilation. J Emerg Med. 2010;38:633–1.
20. Heffener AC, et al. Predictors of the complications of postintubation hypotension during emergency airway management. J Crit Care. 2012;27:587–93.
21. Kim JM, et al. Sedative dose and patient variable impacts on postintubation hypotension in emergency airway management. Am J Emerg Med. 2019;37:1248–53.
22. Kautto H. Attenuation of the circulatory response to laryngoscopy and intubation by fentanyl. Acta Anaesthesiol Scand. 1982;26:217–21.
23. Chen CT, Toung TJK, Donham RT, et al. Fentanyl dosage for suppression of circulatory response to laryngoscopy and endotracheal intubation. Anesthesiol Rev. 1986;13:37–42.
24. Dorsey DP, Joffe AM. Physiologic and pathophysiologic responses to intubation. In: Hagberg CA, Artime CA, Aziz MF, editors. Hagberg and Benumof's Airway management. 4th ed: Elsevier; 2018.
25. Takita K, Morimoto Y, Kemmotsu O. Tracheal lidocaine attenuates the cardiovascular response to endotracheal intubation. Can J Anaesth. 2001;48:732–6.
26. Mirakhur R. Bradycardia with laryngeal spraying in children. Acta Anaesthesiol Scand. 1982;26:130–2.
27. Dorsey DP, Joffe AM. Physiologic and pathophysiologic responses to intubation. In: Hagberg CA, Artime CA, Aziz MF, editors. Hagberg and Benumof's Airway management. 4th ed: Elsevier; 2018.

28. Rotandoet a. Push dose pressors: experience in critically ill patients outside of the operating room. Am J Emerg Med. 2019;37:494–8.
29. Tehrani, B.N. et al. Standardized Team-Based Care for Cardiogenic Shock. J Am Coll Cardiol. 2019;73:1659–1669.
30. van Diepen S, et al. Contemporary Management of Cardiogenic Shock: a Scientific Statement from the American Heart Association. On behalf of the American Heart Association Council on clinical cardiology; council on cardiovascular and stroke nursing; council on quality of care and outcomes research; and Mission: lifeline. Circulation. 2017;136:e232–68.
31. Kim JM, et al. Sedative dose and patient variable impacts on postintubation hypotension in emergency airway management. Am J Emerg Med. 2019;37:1248–53.
32. Gomez H, Pinsky MR. Effect of mechanical ventilation on heart-lung interactions. In: Tobin M, editor. Principles and practice of mechanical ventilation: McGraw Hill; 2013.
33. Venteuolo CE, Klinger JR. Management of acute right ventricular failure in the intensive care unit. Ann Am Thorac Soc. 2014;11:811–22.
34. Horak J, Weiss S. Emergent management of the airway: new pharmacology and the control of comorbidities in cardiac disease, ischemia and valvular disease. Crit Care Clin. 2000;16:411–27.
35. Neumar RW, et al. Part 1: executive summary. American Heart Association guidelines update for cardiopulmonary resuscitation and emergency cardiovascular care. Circulation. 2015;132:S315–67.
36. Hasegawa K, et al. Association of prehospital advanced airway management with neurologic outcome and survival in patients with out-of-hospital cardiac arrest. JAMA. 2013;309:257–66.
37. Andersen LW, et al. For the American Heart Association's get with the guidelines – resuscitation investigators. Association between tracheal intubation during adult in-hospital cardiac arrest and survival. JAMA. 2017;317:494–506.

Chapter 10
The Obese Patient

Bradley A. Dengler

Key Points
- The ramped position should be used for intubation of obese patients.
- Obese patients will have a shorter apnea time than lean patients.
- Two people will be required for bag-mask ventilation to ensure adequate oxygen delivery and ventilation.
- The video laryngoscope provides shorter times to intubation and better views than standard direct laryngoscopy.
- Higher levels of PEEP may be needed to support oxygenation.
- Most medications should be dosed based on total body weight except for ketamine, benzodiazepine infusions, and non-depolarizing neuromuscular blockers.

B. A. Dengler (✉)
Department of Neurosurgery, Walter Reed National Military Medical Center, Bethesda, MD, USA
e-mail: Bradley.a.dengler.mil@mail.mil

© Springer Nature Switzerland AG 2021
R. Garvin (ed.), *Intubating the Critically Ill Patient*,
https://doi.org/10.1007/978-3-030-56813-9_10

Obesity in Numbers

- Rates of obesity and especially morbid obesity continue to increase in the United States and throughout the world.
- The current prevalence of obesity has reached 35% in men and 40% in women [1, 2].
- The definition of obesity by the World Health Organization is a body mass index (BMI) over 30 kg/m² and morbid obesity as a BMI over 40 kg/m² [3].
- There is a correlation between obesity and increased mortality in the intensive care unit [3]. This is likely multifactorial but can at least, in part, be due to the difficulty and challenges obesity places on the respiratory system.
- The emergency physician and intensivist must be prepared and comfortable managing the airway in the obese patient.

Impact of Obesity

Physiology

- Obese patients have a decreased oxygen reserve as a result of collapse of the smaller distal airways and alveoli [3–6].
- This micro-atelectasis leads to a ventilation-perfusion mismatch in the well-perfused distal lung bases and therefore an increase in the alveolar-arterial oxygen gradient [7, 8].
- Placing obese patients supine during the induction phase leads to worsening of the atelectasis and the ventilation–perfusion mismatch [3, 8].
- This worsening ventilation–perfusion mismatch can lead to hypoxia.
- Obese patients also have less of an apneic reserve leading to rapid desaturations with periods of apnea. This is due to the decreasing functional residual capacity (FRC) that occurs with increasing body mass index [3, 9].
- The functional residual capacity can decrease as much as 50% in obese individuals with induction of anesthesia compared to 20% in non-obese individuals [7, 8].

- Excess body fat leads to increased metabolic rates, oxygen consumption, and increased CO_2 production [3, 9–12]. This excess CO_2 production along with decreased FRC and lung volumes lead to obese patients having increased respiratory rates in the range of 15–21 breaths per minute (in comparison to lean individuals at 10–12 breaths per minute) [13, 14].
- Additionally, the micro-atelectasis along with decreased chest wall compliance in the obese patient leads to increased airway resistance which can contribute to difficulty with bag-mask ventilation (BMV).

Pre-intubation

- Pre-intubation set up and evaluation of the patient are the most critical steps in the process of managing a difficult airway to ensure that the provider anticipates challenges and problems before they occur.
- Adequate pre-oxygenation prior to induction is imperative for successful intubation given the diminished apneic reserve in the obese patient.
- Patients should generally be positioned with their head up at least 25 degrees, as this will provide longer periods of apnea without desaturations [7, 18, 19].
- A facemask with a good seal and tidal volume breathing for 3 minutes is the best method of pre-oxygenation in this patient population [7, 20]. Oxygen can also be delivered via nasopharyngeal insufflation after pre-oxygenation, which can extend the apnea time before desaturation occurs to almost 4 minutes [21].
- The use of both continuous positive airway pressure (CPAP) delivered via facemask prior to induction and positive end expiratory pressure (PEEP) after induction can also extend the apnea period and it will help to achieve higher end tidal oxygen content more rapidly [22–24].
- Patients with BMI over 30 kg/m^2, facial hair, obstructive sleep apnea, age greater than 57, and Mallampati Score of

III or IV, are all at risk of having difficult bag-mask ventilation [15, 16].

- In the obese patient, difficulty with bag-mask ventilation is due to redundant supraglottic tissue, poor chest wall compliance, and increased upper airway resistance.
- The ability to provide adequate bag-mask ventilation is vitally important to accomplish in the obese patient given the speed at which obese patients will develop a drop in their oxygen saturation.
- Airway adjuncts such as the oropharyngeal or nasopharyngeal airway can help eliminate the obstruction caused by redundant supraglottic tissues and improve the ability to conduct bag-mask ventilation (BMV).
- A two-person technique is optimal for the BMV of the obese patient: The first provider focuses on getting an adequate seal of the mask while performing a jaw thrust maneuver while the second provider focuses on adequately squeezing the bag with two hands to help overcome the increased airway resistance and decreased chest compliance [3, 17].

Intubation

- Studies are conflicting as to whether there is increased difficulty in accomplishing an endotracheal intubation in the obese patient, but the most recent meta-analysis did not show a significant difference in difficulty between intubations of the obese and lean patient [16].
- Although obesity itself might not be a risk factor for difficult intubation, there is evidence that patients' with increasing BMI or a BMI greater than 30 kg/m^2 will be a difficult intubation [15, 25].
- Other predictors of difficulty with tracheal intubation include neck circumference greater than 43 cm, Mallampati score greater than 3, and poor dentition [26, 27].
- The standard sniffing position for orotracheal intubation has been shown to be less ideal for the obese patient and

lead to increased intubation attempts and time to intubation.

- Instead, the patient should be placed into a ramped position where their external auditory canal is at the same level as their sternal notch (see Chap. 4: Preparing the Patient). This position is easily accomplished by placing multiple folded blankets underneath the head and shoulders [7, 19, 28].

- With the patient positioned appropriately, the next step is to choose the correct intubation devices. There is a slight trend toward better visualization, decreased attempts, and decreased time to intubation with the video laryngoscope versus direct laryngoscopy with a Macintosh Laryngoscope [3, 13, 29–34].

- The bougie is an useful adjunct in obese patients with redundant tissue causing only the epiglottis or epiglottis and partial arytenoids to be visualized during direct laryngoscopy.

- The laryngeal mask airway (LMA) and intubating laryngeal mask airway (ILMA) are also very useful rescue devices for the difficult-to-intubate obese patient. These devices have been successful in both lean and obese patients in oxygenating and ventilating a patient after failed attempts of direct laryngoscopy. These devices are also able to oxygenate and ventilate even when there is a poor grade view on direct laryngoscopy [3, 35, 36].

- An ILMA can allow an endotracheal tube to be passed through the laryngeal device at a later time to obtain a definitive airway. This procedure has been shown to be up to 96% effective in obese patients with only a slightly longer time to intubation [35].

- The fall back of using a fiberoptic scope might be more challenging in the obese patient because the redundant oropharyngeal tissue collapses around the fiberoptic scope, making it difficult to see the appropriate anatomy.

- A novel technique is to place an LMA or ILMA to maintain ventilation and oxygenation and then pass a bronchoscope along with an intubating catheter through the supraglottic airway device. The intubating catheter can remain in place while the supraglottic device and the bronchoscope are withdrawn. This will then allow an endotracheal tube to be passed over the intubating catheter and securing the airway [7, 37–39].

Post-intubation

- Confirmation that the endotracheal tube is in the trachea and has not been misplaced into the esophagus is essential.
- The usual methods of confirming tube position such as auscultation and watching for chest rise and fall might be difficult due to the patient's body habitus.
- The chest X-ray may be more difficult to interpret due to the excessive subcutaneous fat.
- Pulse oximetry readings might be low or abnormal due to excess soft tissue on the fingers or earlobes.
- Capnography and disposable carbon dioxide detectors are likely the best options for confirming correct placement of the endotracheal tube in this patient population [3, 40, 41].

Mechanical Ventilation

- Once the patient is intubated, placing the obese ventilated patient in the reverse Trendelenberg position, or with their head of bed elevated will help to improve pulmonary mechanics and oxygenation [3, 42].
- The tidal volumes on the ventilator should be set to 6–8 cc/kg of *ideal body weight*. The patient's total body weight should not be used as this will substantially overestimate the tidal volume [3, 13].
- As discussed above, the use of PEEP is beneficial in obese patients, as it will help to recruit and stent open atelectatic airways, and a PEEP of 10 cm H_2O in these patients has been shown to provide improved oxygenation [3, 43].

- Obese patients produce more CO_2 than lean patients due to their increased mass, resulting in a more rapid shallow breathing pattern, thus a higher initial respiratory rate should be set on the ventilator [13, 14, 44].
- There have been no definitive studies completed to determine the best ventilation mode in these patients but there are some data to support that obese patients may do better with pressure support ventilation and have less post-extubation pulmonary complications with this mode compared to others [14, 45].

Medications

- The dosing of medications for intubation in the obese patient can be challenging as the lipophilicity and hydrophilicity of medications can change their effect on the patient given the large amount of fat.
- There is a substantial literature to support that when using succinylcholine it should be dosed at 1 mg/kg of total body weight, as this will allow for the best laryngoscopic view [3, 12, 46, 47].
- Non-depolarizing neuromuscular blockers in contrast should be dosed by ideal body weight [12, 47, 48].
- Induction agents become slightly more challenging because medications such as propofol and etomidate are lipophilic, thus their volume of distribution will be elevated in obese individuals. This elevated volume of distribution requires dosing based on total body weight.
- Depending on the clinical circumstance, a dose of propofol less than what the total body weight calls for might be ideal given its propensity for cardiovascular depression at higher doses [48–50].
- Benzodiazepines are also in the lipophilic category and should therefore be dosed based on total body weight.
- During continuous infusions, the benzodiazepines should be titrated down closer to ideal body weight dosages to prevent excess build up in the adipose tissue [12, 49, 51, 52].

- Ketamine has been shown to be most effectively dosed according to lean body mass. Lean body mass is estimated by adding 20% to the ideal body weight [3, 53].

References

1. Flegal KM, Kruszon-Moran D, Carroll MD, Fryar CD, Ogden CL. Trends in obesity among adults in the United States, 2005 to 2014. JAMA. 2016;315(21):2284–91.
2. Richardson AS, Chen C, Sturm R, Azhar G, Miles J, Larkin J, et al. Obesity prevention interventions and implications for energy balance in the United States and Mexico: a systematic review of the evidence and meta-analysis. Obesity (Silver Spring, MD). 2019;27(9):1390–403.
3. Dargin J, Medzon R. Emergency department management of the airway in obese adults. Ann Emerg Med. 2010;56(2):95–104.
4. Steier J, Lunt A, Hart N, Polkey MI, Moxham J. Observational study of the effect of obesity on lung volumes. Thorax. 2014;69(8):752–9.
5. El-Solh A, Sikka P, Bozkanat E, Jaafar W, Davies J. Morbid obesity in the medical ICU. Chest. 2001;120(6):1989–97.
6. Marik P, Varon J. The obese patient in the ICU. Chest. 1998;113(2):492–8.
7. Murphy C, Wong DT. Airway management and oxygenation in obese patients. Can J Anaesth. 2013;60(9):929–45.
8. Pelosi P, Croci M, Ravagnan I, Tredici S, Pedoto A, Lissoni A, et al. The effects of body mass on lung volumes, respiratory mechanics, and gas exchange during general anesthesia. Anesth Analg. 1998;87(3):654–60.
9. Adams JP, Murphy PG. Obesity in anaesthesia and intensive care. Br J Anaesth. 2000;85(1):91–108.
10. Kuchta KF. Pathophysiologic changes of obesity. Anesthesiol Clin North Am. 2005;23(3):421–9. vi
11. Luce JM. Respiratory complications of obesity. Chest. 1980;78(4):626–31.
12. Ogunnaike BO, Jones SB, Jones DB, Provost D, Whitten CW. Anesthetic considerations for bariatric surgery. Anesth Analg. 2002;95(6):1793–805.
13. Parker BK, Manning S, Winters ME. The crashing obese patient. West J Emerg Med. 2019;20(2):323–30.

14. De Jong A, Chanques G, Jaber S. Mechanical ventilation in obese ICU patients: from intubation to extubation. Crit Care. 2017;21(1):63.
15. Langeron O, Birenbaum A, Le Sache F, Raux M. Airway management in obese patient. Minerva Anestesiol 2014;80(3):382–392.
16. Moon TS, Fox PE, Somasundaram A, Minhajuddin A, Gonzales MX, Pak TJ, et al. The influence of morbid obesity on difficult intubation and difficult mask ventilation. J Anesth. 2019;33(1):96–102.
17. Langeron O, Masso E, Huraux C, Guggiari M, Bianchi A, Coriat P, et al. Prediction of difficult mask ventilation. Anesthesiology. 2000;92(5):1229–36.
18. Dixon BJ, Dixon JB, Carden JR, Burn AJ, Schachter LM, Playfair JM, et al. Preoxygenation is more effective in the 25 degrees head-up position than in the supine position in severely obese patients: a randomized controlled study. Anesthesiology. 2005;102(6):1110–5; discussion 5A.
19. Boyce JR, Ness T, Castroman P, Gleysteen JJ. A preliminary study of the optimal anesthesia positioning for the morbidly obese patient. Obes Surg. 2003;13(1):4–9.
20. Benumof JL. Preoxygenation: best method for both efficacy and efficiency. Anesthesiology. 1999;91(3):603–5.
21. Baraka AS, Taha SK, Siddik-Sayyid SM, Kanazi GE, El-Khatib MF, Dagher CM, et al. Supplementation of pre-oxygenation in morbidly obese patients using nasopharyngeal oxygen insufflation. Anaesthesia. 2007;62(8):769–73.
22. Coussa M, Proietti S, Schnyder P, Frascarolo P, Suter M, Spahn DR, et al. Prevention of atelectasis formation during the induction of general anesthesia in morbidly obese patients. Anesth Analg. 2004;98(5):1491–5, table of contents.
23. Gander S, Frascarolo P, Suter M, Spahn DR, Magnusson L. Positive end-expiratory pressure during induction of general anesthesia increases duration of nonhypoxic apnea in morbidly obese patients. Anesth Analg. 2005;100(2):580–4.
24. Delay JM, Sebbane M, Jung B, Nocca D, Verzilli D, Pouzeratte Y, et al. The effectiveness of noninvasive positive pressure ventilation to enhance preoxygenation in morbidly obese patients: a randomized controlled study. Anesth Analg. 2008;107(5):1707–13.
25. Lundstrom LH, Moller AM, Rosenstock C, Astrup G, Wetterslev J. High body mass index is a weak predictor for difficult and failed tracheal intubation: a cohort study of 91,332 consecutive

patients scheduled for direct laryngoscopy registered in the Danish anesthesia database. Anesthesiology. 2009;110(2):266–74.

26. Gonzalez H, Minville V, Delanoue K, Mazerolles M, Concina D, Fourcade O. The importance of increased neck circumference to intubation difficulties in obese patients. Anesth Analg. 2008;106(4):1132–6, table of contents.

27. Brodsky JB, Lemmens HJ, Brock-Utne JG, Vierra M, Saidman LJ. Morbid obesity and tracheal intubation. Anesth Analg. 2002;94(3):732–6; table of contents.

28. Collins JS, Lemmens HJ, Brodsky JB, Brock-Utne JG, Levitan RM. Laryngoscopy and morbid obesity: a comparison of the "sniff" and "ramped" positions. Obes Surg. 2004;14(9):1171–5.

29. Yumul R, Elvir-Lazo OL, White PF, Sloninsky A, Kaplan M, Kariger R, et al. Comparison of three video laryngoscopy devices to direct laryngoscopy for intubating obese patients: a randomized controlled trial. J Clin Anesth. 2016;31:71–7.

30. Ander F, Magnuson A, Berggren L, Ahlstrand R, de Leon A. Time-to-intubation in obese patients. A randomized study comparing direct laryngoscopy and video laryngoscopy in experienced anesthetists. Minerva Anestesiol 2017;83(9):906–913.

31. Dhonneur G, Abdi W, Ndoko SK, Amathieu R, Risk N, El Housseini L, et al. Video-assisted versus conventional tracheal intubation in morbidly obese patients. Obes Surg. 2009;19(8):1096–101.

32. Cooper RM, Pacey JA, Bishop MJ, McCluskey SA. Early clinical experience with a new video laryngoscope (GlideScope) in 728 patients. Can J Anaesth. 2005;52(2):191–8.

33. Marrel J, Blanc C, Frascarolo P, Magnusson L. Video laryngoscopy improves intubation condition in morbidly obese patients. Eur J Anaesthesiol. 2007;24(12):1045–9.

34. Dhonneur G, Ndoko S, Amathieu R, Housseini LE, Poncelet C, Tual L. Tracheal intubation using the Airtraq® in morbid obese patients undergoing emergency cesarean delivery. Anesthesiology. 2007;106(3):629–30.

35. Frappier J, Guenoun T, Journois D, Philippe H, Aka E, Cadi P, et al. Airway management using the intubating laryngeal mask airway for the morbidly obese patient. Anesth Analg. 2003;96(5):1510–5, table of contents.

36. Keller C, Brimacombe J, Kleinsasser A, Brimacombe L. The Laryngeal Mask Airway ProSeal(TM) as a temporary ventilatory device in grossly and morbidly obese patients before

laryngoscope-guided tracheal intubation. Anesth Analg. 2002;94(3):737–40; table of contents.

37. Cook TM, Seller C, Gupta K, Thornton M, O'Sullivan E. Non-conventional uses of the Aintree intubating catheter in management of the difficult airway. Anaesthesia. 2007;62(2):169–74.

38. Berkow LC, Schwartz JM, Kan K, Corridore M, Heitmiller ES. Use of the laryngeal mask airway-Aintree intubating catheter-fiberoptic bronchoscope technique for difficult intubation. J Clin Anesth. 2011;23(7):534–9.

39. Combes X, Sauvat S, Leroux B, Dumerat M, Sherrer E, Motamed C, et al. Intubating laryngeal mask airway in morbidly obese and lean patients: a comparative study. Anesthesiology. 2005;102(6):1106–9; discussion 5A.

40. Brunette DD. Resuscitation of the morbidly obese patient. Am J Emerg Med. 2004;22(1):40–7.

41. Mort TC. Esophageal intubation with indirect clinical tests during emergency tracheal intubation: a report on patient morbidity. J Clin Anesth. 2005;17(4):255–62.

42. Perilli V, Sollazzi L, Bozza P, Modesti C, Chierichini A, Tacchino RM, et al. The effects of the reverse Trendelenburg position on respiratory mechanics and blood gases in morbidly obese patients during bariatric surgery. Anesth Analg. 2000;91(6):1520–5.

43. Pelosi P, Ravagnan I, Giurati G, Panigada M, Bottino N, Tredici S, et al. Positive end-expiratory pressure improves respiratory function in obese but not in normal subjects during anesthesia and paralysis. Anesthesiology. 1999;91(5):1221–31.

44. Chlif M, Keochkerian D, Choquet D, Vaidie A, Ahmaidi S. Effects of obesity on breathing pattern, ventilatory neural drive and mechanics. Respir Physiol Neurobiol. 2009;168(3):198–202.

45. Zoremba M, Kalmus G, Dette F, Kuhn C, Wulf H. Effect of intraoperative pressure support vs pressure controlled ventilation on oxygenation and lung function in moderately obese adults. Anaesthesia. 2010;65(2):124–9.

46. Lemmens HJ, Brodsky JB. The dose of succinylcholine in morbid obesity. Anesth Analg. 2006;102(2):438–42.

47. Freid EB. The rapid sequence induction revisited: obesity and sleep apnea syndrome. Anesthesiol Clin North Am. 2005;23(3):551–64. viii

48. Passannante AN, Tielborg M. Anesthetic management of patients with obesity with and without sleep apnea. Clin Chest Med. 2009;30(3):569–79. x

49. Pieracci FM, Barie PS, Pomp A. Critical care of the bariatric patient. Crit Care Med. 2006;34(6):1796–804.

50. Servin F, Farinotti R, Haberer JP, Desmonts JM. Propofol infusion for maintenance of anesthesia in morbidly obese patients receiving nitrous oxide. A clinical and pharmacokinetic study. Anesthesiology. 1993;78(4):657–65.
51. Greenblatt DJ, Abernethy DR, Locniskar A, Harmatz JS, Limjuco RA, Shader RI. Effect of age, gender, and obesity on midazolam kinetics. Anesthesiology. 1984;61(1):27–35.
52. Erstad BL. Dosing of medications in morbidly obese patients in the intensive care unit setting. Intensive Care Med. 2004;30(1):18–32.
53. Wulfsohn NL. Ketamine dosage for induction based on lean body mass. Anesth Analg. 1972;51(2):299-305.

Chapter 11
Intubating the Neurologically Injured Patient

Shaheryar Hafeez

Key Points
- Airway protection is the most common reason patients with neurologic injury require intubation.
- Cerebral perfusion pressure (CPP) = MAP – ICP; ICP >20 mmHg is likely abnormal.
- Maintaining adequate cerebral and spinal perfusion is crucial in patients with neurologic injury.
- Positioning may need to be altered based on pathophysiology.
- A pre-intubation neurologic exam is crucial prior to airway placement.

S. Hafeez (✉)
Department of Neurosurgery,
UT Health San Antonio, San Antonio, TX, USA
e-mail: Hafeez@uthscsa.edu

© Springer Nature Switzerland AG 2021
R. Garvin (ed.), *Intubating the Critically Ill Patient*,
https://doi.org/10.1007/978-3-030-56813-9_11

Indications for Intubation

Failure to protect the airway can occur due to acute coma, inability to control oral secretions due to neuromuscular disease or cranial neuropathy, cerebral herniation syndrome, and acute cervical spinal cord injury (SCI) [4].

**Prior to intubation: A good neurologic exam is vital prior to intubation to have a basis for comparison.

- Perform a rapid neurological exam
  - Glasgow Coma Scale (GCS)
  - Pupils, facial symmetry, cough/gag, and corneal reflexes
  - Motor function in the face, arms, and legs
  - Assess for gross sensation throughout and locate sensory level if present
  - Tone and reflexes
  - Assess for seizure activity

Acute Stroke, Intracerebral Hemorrhage (ICH), and Aneurysmal Subarachnoid Hemorrhage (SAH)

- Goals:
  - Maintenance of adequate cerebral perfusion pressure is crucial to mitigating secondary brain injury (minimum >60 mmHg).
  - These patients often have poor cerebral autoregulation and any degree of hypotension could cause disastrous ischemic effects on cerebral tissue [4].
- **Pearls:
  - Acute stroke and new onset atrial fibrillation
    The reflex sympathetic response and direct laryngeal reflex may induce rapid ventricular rate and subsequent hemodynamic instability.
  - In SAH, consider the use of nebulized lidocaine in order to protect against the direct laryngeal reflex potentially raising ICP and re-rupture an unsecured aneurysm.

- *Induction agents*: Hemodynamically neutral agents such as etomidate

  Ketamine can also be a good choice to avoid drops in blood pressure.

  What to avoid: Large bolus doses of propofol due to its cardiodepressant effect.

  Considerations: Intravenous lidocaine or beta blockade for cardioprotection prior to induction.
- *Paralytics*: succinylcholine or rocuronium.
- *Technique*: Conventional direct visualization via direct or video laryngoscopy is a reasonable method to consider. Fiberoptic intubation can be considered, but generally, these patients will not be awake or able to cooperate.
- Extra care in patients who receive thrombolytics. Process of laryngoscopy can precipitate bleeding, which could make airway management more difficult.

Traumatic Brain Injury (TBI)

- Goals:
  - TBI patients are trauma patients first and distraction by other injuries may cause unnecessary delays in care and hypoxia.
  - It is important to follow ATLS guidelines when considering intubation of these patients.
  - Patients with acute spinal cord injury (SCI) can also have a TBI and hemodynamic changes from SCI – neurogenic shock – can have tremendous negative consequences for the injured brain that is starving for oxygen and nutrients.
- *Induction agents*:
  - Hemodynamically neutral agents such as etomidate.
  - Ketamine can be useful in helping to maintain CPP.
  - Despite sympathomimetic effects, ketamine is not contraindicated in TBI patients.
- *Paralytics*: succinylcholine or rocuronium [5].

Intubation Methods

Intubation of the patient *without* elevated ICP

- Technique: Rapid sequence intubation.
  - Conventional direct visualization via laryngoscopy or video laryngoscopy are reasonable methods to consider.
  - Fiberoptic intubation may be used as well but generally these patients will not be awake or cooperative.
  - Neck extension is reasonable (unless elevated ICP or cervical spine injury is suspected).
  - **Special Considerations: Focus on maintaining cerebral perfusion pressure (CPP) > 60 mmHg. CPP = MAP – ICP.

Intubation of the patient *with* elevated ICP:

- In severe brain injury with poor neurologic exam – assume ICP is elevated!
- Elevate the HOB. One of the most common mistakes made in intubation of the patient with severe TBI is laying the body flat and performing a neck extension to get the airway secure.
- Intubation with the head flat can cause an increase of approximately 5 cm H_2O in patients with severe TBI [6].
- Intubation should optimally be performed with the head of bed elevated at 30–45 degrees; reverse trendelenburg can also be used
- Cerebral perfusion pressure target:
  - If invasive ICP monitor is present – aim for CPP >60.
  - If invasive ICP monitor is NOT present – assume ICP is 20 and adjust MAP to maintain CPP >60.
- **Pearl: For a patient in the trauma bay with an acute severe TBI who has signs of elevated intracranial pressure or cerebral herniation syndrome, consider an upright or *tomahawk intubation*.
- Position yourself in front of the patient with a video laryngoscope.
- Pull the glottis and epiglottis toward you.
- Insert tube from above or on elevated platform [7]

Spinal Cord Injury and Acute Neuromuscular Failure

- Goals: Patients with a high cervical cord spinal cord injury oftentimes require mechanical ventilation because they do not have innervation to provide spontaneous respirations.
- Injuries down to T6 will result in loss of accessory muscle use.
- Patients with SCI are also trauma patients and all ATLS protocols must be considered.
- According to one study, SCI patients present with concomitant TBI up to 60% of the time [8].
- Special considerations:
  1. High cervical spinal cord injury without lung pathology
     - Ineffective respirations
     - Weak cough
     - Paradoxical breathing
  2. High cervical spinal cord injury WITH primary lung pathology
     Patients with acute lung injury – aspiration pneumonitis, pulmonary embolism, and pulmonary contusions:
     - Decreased vital capacity
     - V/Q mismatch
     - Inflammation
     - Pleural effusions and edema
- Induction agents:
  - If a patient is in neurogenic shock, consider hemodynamically neutral agents such as ketamine and etomidate.
  - In patients with shock, catecholamine depletion may have occurred, in which case, ketamine can have negative inotropic effects [10].
  - Induction medications to avoid: propofol.
  - A decrease in spinal cord perfusion pressure could lead to spinal cord ischemia.
  - While there is a still debate over whether high MAP goals are beneficial in SCI, hypotension is associated with decreased recovery and stagnant ASIA scores [11]
- Technique:

- Awake fiberoptic intubation is the preferred approach for patients with high cervical SCI.
- This permits video visualization of the airway without neck extension and can allow for preservation of the neurologic exam [9].
- Care and considerations must be given to avoid extension of the neck.
- There is a natural tendency during intubation to extend the neck and sometimes elevate the head off the bed to extend the neck further for optimal visualization.
- These techniques are contraindicated as further neck mobilization can cause secondary injury of the spinal cord.
- Providing manual in-line stabilization is preferred.

Neurocritical Care Checklist Questions

- Why is this patient being intubated?
- Is there a suspicion of elevated ICP?
- What is our MAP goal based on calculated CPP?
- Does the patient have or require spinal precautions?
- Is seizure activity present?
- What hemodynamically neutral medications are we using?
- Has a neuro exam been performed prior to induction and paralytics?

References

1. Cole CD, Gottfried ON, Gupta DK, Couldwell WT. Total intravenous anesthesia: advantages for intracranial surgery. Neurosurgery. 2007;61:369–77.
2. Grathwohl KW, Black IH, Spinella PC, et al. Total intravenous anesthesia including ketamine versus volatile gas anesthesia for combat-related operative traumatic brain injury. Anesthesiology. 2008;109:44–53.
3. Engelhard K, Werner C, Mollenberg O, et al. Effects of remifentanil/propofol in comparison with isoflurane on dynamic cere-

brovascular autoregulation in humans. Acta Anaesthesiol Scand. 2001;45:9971–6.

4. Tang SC, Huang YW, Shieh JS, Huang SJ, Yip PK, Jeng JS. Dynamic cerebral autoregulation in carotid stenosis before and after carotid stenting. J Vasc Surg. 2008;48(1):88–92.

5. Seder DB, Riker RR, Jagoda A, Smith WS, Weingart SD. Emergency neurological life support: airway, ventilation, and sedation. Neurocrit Care. 2012;

6. Feldman Z, Kanter MJ, Robertson CS, Contant CF, Hayes C, Sheinberg MA, et al. Effect of head elevation on intracranial pressure, cerebral perfusion pressure, and cerebral blood flow in head-injured patients. J Neurosurg. 1992;76(2):207–11.

7. Choi HY, Oh YM, Kang GH, et al. A randomized comparison simulating face to face endotracheal intubation of Pentax airway scope, C-MAC video laryngoscope, Glidescope video laryngoscope, and Macintosh laryngoscope. Biomed Res Int. 2015;2015:961782.

8. Macciocchi S, Seel RT, Warshowsky A, Thompson N, Barlow K. Co-occurring traumatic brain injury and acute spinal cord injury rehabilitation outcomes. Arch Phys Med Rehabil. 2012;93(10):1788–94.

9. Austin N, Krishnamoorthy V, Dagal A. Airway management in cervical spine injury. Int J CritIllnInj Sci. 2014;4(1):50–6.

10. Dewhirst E, Frazier WJ, Leder M, Fraser DD, Tobias JD. Cardiac arrest following ketamine administration for rapid sequence intubation. J Intensive Care Med. 2013;28(6):375–9.

11. Ryken TC, et al. Guidelines for the management of acute cervical spine and SCI. The acute cardiopulmonary management of patients with cervical spinal cord injuries. Neurosurgery. 2013;

Chapter 12
Intubating the Septic Patient: Avoiding the Crash and Burn

Rahul K. Shah

> **Key Points**
> - Septic patients are physiologically challenged and therefore require specialized management.
> - Pre-oxygenation is essential to avoid cardiovascular collapse.
> - Patients require preemptive resuscitation and ongoing sepsis treatment.
> - Choice and dose of induction and paralytic agents are critical to ensure further compromise does not occur.

Why Intubating the Septic Patient Is a Challenge?

Septic patients rob intensivists of their greatest ally: TIME! contributing issues to airway management in a septic patient:

R. K. Shah (✉)
Department of Neurology/ Neuro Critical Care, Bakersfield Memorial Hospital, Bakersfield, CA, USA

© Springer Nature Switzerland AG 2021   115
R. Garvin (ed.), *Intubating the Critically Ill Patient*,
https://doi.org/10.1007/978-3-030-56813-9_12

- Pre-oxygenation is far less effective in septic patients and they typically do not tolerate any level of apnea, mainly due to significant physiological compromise with ventilation/perfusion (V/Q) abnormalities and poor functional residual capacities [1].
- Unstable hemodynamic status combined with sedatives and raised intrathoracic pressure can often worsen hypotension and make the process of airway management even more tricky.
- There is limited evidence to suggest that a certain induction agent and sedative will work appropriately on all septic patients.
- Each patient requires a personalized assessment for the optimal combination of drugs depending on their vital status and underlying pathophysiology.

Timing: Earlier Is Better

- The chapter "When to Pull the Trigger" details the factors to consider when making the crucial decision of when to intubate.
- Knowing when to pull the trigger in septic patients can be complex as they can decompensate rapidly.
- Early identification of clinical signs and indices leading to a preemptive, early intubation, may turn out to be the difference between intubating a patient in a fairly controlled manner vs doing a crash airway in a severely hemodynamically compromised patient [1, 2].
- *If your patient can be intubated with little or no sedation because of effects of sepsis, you have waited too long* [1, 2, 3].

Pre-Oxygenation

- *ICU patients may desaturate below 85% saturated oxygen in arterial blood (SPO₂) in less than 23 secs, which is almost 25 times faster than healthy individuals* [1, 40, 41].

- *This time is even shorter in patients with septic shock once spontaneous breathing efforts stop after administration of paralytics.*
- Pre-oxygenation helps to increase alveolar O_2 reserve and in turn increases apnea time – the duration between cessation of breathing to desaturation (typically below SPO_2 90%).
- *The time to desaturation can be doubled by increasing the FIO_2 from 90% to 100% [34, 35].*
- Multiple studies have highlighted the benefit of using NIPPV for pre-oxygenation over standard bag-valve ventilation in the critically ill population.
- NIPPV with positive end expiratory pressure (PEEP) assists in increasing the mean airway pressure and enhanced recruitment of alveoli.
- *In a randomized clinical trial, Baillard et al. showed a significant reduction in the number of patients desaturating at 3 mins using NIPPV versus standard pre-oxygenation with a bag valve mask (7% vs 46%) [35].*
- The NO DESAT technique, also known as apneic oxygenation, wherein a nasal cannula continues to deliver O_2 at 15 L/min during laryngoscopy is now commonly used across many EDs and ICUs.
- Transnasal humidified rapid insufflation ventilatory exchange (THRIVE) allows for providing 60–70 L of humidified O_2 during the same period and has the advantage of prolonging the apnea time over traditional techniques while providing some degree of CO_2 clearance, delaying a critical rise in CO_2 concentration [35, 36].
- Although widely used, SpO_2 and blood gas indices are not the most accurate at assessing efficacy of pre- oxygenation since they are affected by cardiorespiratory interactions [1].
- *End tidal O_2 (ETO_2) concentration when available, should be the preferred index to use. We define adequate pre-oxygenation as an $ETO_2 > = 90\%$ [1, 37–39].*
- *Although there are no randomized studies comparing these techniques specifically in the septic population, any intervention that helps increase the O_2 reserve and prolongs apnea time in this unique ICU population will be beneficial [35].*

Ongoing Sepsis Management

It is essential to continue aggressive sepsis treatment while addressing the airway. Proper resuscitation efforts can aid in ensuring a far smoother intubation. It is beyond the scope of this chapter to discuss sepsis management in its entirety but we have summarized some of the important components of sepsis management that if properly addressed, may aid in safer airway management:

- *Hypothermia*
  - Hypothermia in a septic patient is an independent predictor of higher mortality [4, 5].
  - Immediate correction of hypothermia using surface warmers is extremely important.
  - Correcting hypothermia could potentially aid in decreasing pressor requirement, improving effectiveness of resuscitation efforts.
  - Surface warmers like bear huggers, heating pads, Arctic Sun, or infusion of warm IV fluids may be used.
- *Acidemia*
  - Bicarbonate pushes have been utilized prior to intubating to either improve hemodynamics so that that the patient tolerates sedatives better or to decrease overall pressor requirement.
  - This is purely anecdotal with no evidence to support it.
  - *The surviving sepsis guidelines recommend against the use of bicarbonate in patients with pH > 7.15 for the above indication for patients with hypoperfusion-induced lactic acidemia* [6].
  - Goal is to correct the underlying acidemia.
- *Hypotension*
  - Adequate fluid resuscitation forms the core of sepsis management and could potentially prevent the need for pressors.
  - Optimize fluid resuscitation based on patient's fluid responsiveness, using dynamic markers such as pulse pressure or stroke volume variation, ultrasound evaluation, etc.

- Pressors can be started while fluid resuscitation is in progress to prevent amount of time spent with MAP <65 mmHg to decrease risk of end-organ damage.
- *Norepinephrine is the recommended first choice pressor in sepsis* [6, 7].
- Vasopressin or epinephrine are good second-line agent that can be added as adjuncts to or decrease the dose of norepinephrine [6].
- When using epinephrine, lactate clearance as a guide to resuscitation may be inaccurate as it may cause increased lactate production by stimulating skeletal muscle beta-2 adrenergic receptors.
- Dobutamine should be reserved for patients with persistent hypoperfusion in spite of adequate fluid resuscitation and high norepinephrine doses [6, 7].
- *Patients with poor cardiac output not just from sepsis but from underlying cardiac dysfunction are typically the ideal candidates for an inotropic agent like dopamine* [6, 7].

Equipment/Technique-Related Issues

- *Preparation*

Chapters 3, 4, and 5 cover in depth the preparation needed prior to intubation in the ED and ICU including answers to common questions regarding equipment, etc.

- Every critically ill patient and by default every septic patient must be considered as a difficult airway (DA) as you will typically not have the luxury of much preparation time.

It is essential when available, to have video laryngoscope as well as an advanced airway kit available bedside prior to making the first intubation attempt [1].

- An intubation checklist which involves a clear delineation of duties within the team involved, including a second intubating physician available bedside, if the first attempt fails, is suggested.

- *Bag-Valve Mask (BVM) Ventilation*
  - Septic patients are a very high-aspiration risk, due to excessive secretions, altered level of consciousness, and delayed gastric emptying.
  - Aggressive BVM ventilation in these patients can increase the risk of aspiration, and should be avoided if possible [1, 8].
  - BVM ventilation in patients with septic shock also runs the risk of worsening hypotension by decreasing venous return abruptly [1].
  - *Low volume, low steady rate of face mask ventilation is preferred* [1, 8].

- *Endotracheal (ET) Tube*
  - When intubating a patient in septic shock, the first look quite often is the only look one gets to intubate in these patients.
  - It is very common to encounter glottic and supraglottic edema secondary to systemic inflammatory response syndrome (SIRS) or even previous intubations.
  - *Consider using a smaller diameter ET tube like a 7 Fr or smaller or at least have them prepped and ready before attempting the first pass with a larger tube.*
  - The major downside in using a smaller ET tube is that bronchoscopy becomes more difficult.
  - However, securing the airway and stabilizing the patient should always be your foremost priority even if a smaller tube is required.

Drugs

Etomidate

- Etomidate is often considered the most ideal induction agent as it is extremely lipophilic and crosses the blood-brain barrier rapidly resulting in very quick onset of action.

- It does not cause hypotension and is favorable on hemodynamics which is why it is the first-choice induction agent in most cases of intubation in the ED and ICU.
- There are some concerns regarding its use in the septic patient [1, 11–13].
  - *Adrenal Suppression*

    Several studies have confirmed etomidate's inhibition of 11 beta-hydroxylase resulting in transient adrenal suppression [1, 6, 14–18].

    Although this suppression is transient, it is unclear exactly how long the suppression persists, literature reports between 24 and 72 hrs.

    More recent reports suggest that in septic patients with decreased hepatic metabolism and poor renal clearance, the duration may be longer [17–19].
  - *Effects on Mortality*

    There is no clear consensus, and herein lies the major topic of contention with literature showing mixed results [14, 16, 18, 20].

    Two meta-analysis by Chan et al. and Albert et al. among others showed increased mortality in septic patients where etomidate was used but both studies had some obvious limitations, smaller sample size, and majority of the included studies being single center and observational in nature [16, 18].

    The meta-analysis by Gu et al. published in CHEST in 2015, thus far the largest and most extensive of meta-analysis looking at single dose etomidate for induction and association with outcomes, did not find any increased mortality in patients receiving etomidate for induction [14].
  - Etomidate with Steroids

    Some studies have looked at groups receiving steroids with etomidate vs etomidate alone, and as yet have shown no clear evidence of improved outcomes.
  - The *surviving* sepsis guidelines do not recommend adding steroids for that purpose [6, 21].

- Although some experts have proposed discontinuing the use of etomidate for induction in septic patients, there is no official consensus on whether using etomidate actually worsens outcomes.

Ketamine

- One of the drugs that has been getting a lot more attention recently as an ideal RSI agent in the critically ill is ketamine.
- Ketamine has a lot of properties that make it an ideal agent for the hemodynamically compromised patient.
- Quick onset of action, short acting, induces free radical scavenging, bronchodilatation, NMDA blocking properties resulting in analgesia, and most importantly, propensity to increase blood pressure and heart rate [1, 10, 17, 22–24].

For years, concerns that ketamine caused raised intracranial pressure (ICP) precluded its use in traumatic brain injury or other neuro patients. However, multiple recent studies have debunked this theory [10, 11, 13, 23–25].

- Ketamine is now believed to augment cerebral perfusion without increasing ICP.
- Its use should be avoided in patients with preexisting/ ongoing ischemic cardiomyopathy due to its sympathomimetic properties [10].
- If the patient does not have any obvious contraindications, ketamine can be considered a safe and effective option as an induction agent.

Propofol

- Propofol can cause hypotension and bradycardia, limiting its use in the hemodynamically unstable septic patient.
- *In the setting of sepsis/septic shock with varying levels of depressed mental status as well as poor hepatic clearance,*

desired levels of sedation can be achieved by using half the dose of propofol at 0.25 mg/kg or 0.5 mg/kg compared to the standard 1–2 mg/kg, hence potentially ameliorating the likelihood of causing profound hypotension and bradycardia.

- Propofol's short-acting properties and the familiarity that many providers have with the agent support its use but must be used with caution in this patient population [26].

Remifentanil

- Remifentanil, an ultra-fast-acting opioid, is fast gaining popularity as an analgesic agent for induction and maintenance of anesthesia, both, by itself or in combination with other sedatives to decrease their side effects [10].
- Onset of action is about 1 min and its effects dissociate within 3–10 mins of discontinuation of the infusion.
- It does not need a significant dose adjustment in patients with renal or liver dysfunction.
- It is primarily used in the OR, but all the abovementioned properties make it a very attractive sedative option in the septic patient population in the ICU.
- Further studies are necessary to assess its efficacy and safety in this population though [10].

Novel agents such as carboetomidate and cyclopropyl methoxycarbonyl etomidate carry excellent hemodynamic profile of etomidate but are significantly less potent adrenal suppressants making them extremely attractive options for the future in the septic population [27].

Neuromuscular Blocking Agents (NMBA)

- *Multiple studies have shown the benefit of using NMBA for intubation, especially in the critical care population [11, 28–30].*
- Use of NMBA has been shown to:

- Allow lower dose of sedation reducing degree of resultant hypotension
- Decrease the number of intubation attempts, a sensitive marker for airway-related mortality in the ICU
- Improve bag-mask ventilation and chest-wall compliance
- Overall decrease in the incidence of intubation failure [9, 28–30]

- *Succinylcholine (SC) and, in the last decade or so, rocuronium have been the drugs of choice for RSI* [9, 31, 32]. However, more providers are moving away from SC in recent times, due to the following:
  - The risk of oftentimes fatal hyperkalemia and malignant hyperthermia, more common in the septic, ICU population due to prolonged immobility.
  - In one study, patients receiving SC desaturated 116 secs faster than with rocuronium due to increased muscle activity resulting in greater O_2 consumption [33]. This can be critical in a septic patient with already depleted O_2 reserve [33].
  - In case of a failed first attempt, the extremely short duration of action then becomes a problem, as one may have to wait for effects to wear off and then re-dose, losing precious time [9].

- *Though there is no clear evidence of one NMBA being superior over the other, with the easy availability of the reversal agent Sugammadex in most hospitals now, Rocuronium is fast becoming the preferred NMBA for RSI in critically ill, septic patients* [9, 33].

References

1. Higgs A. Airway management in intensive care medicine. In: Hagberg C, Aziz M, Artime C, editors. Benumof and Hagberg's airway management E-book. 4th ed. Philadelphia, PA: Elsevier Health Sciences; 2018. p. 50580–3192.
2. Delbove A, Darreau C, Hamel JF, Asfar P, Lerolle N. Impact of endotracheal intubation on septic shock outcome: a post hoc analysis of the SEPSISPAM trial. J Crit Care. 2015;30(6):1174–8.

3. de Montmollin E, Aboab J, Ferrer R, Azoulay E, Annane D. Criteria for initiation of invasive ventilation in septic shock: an international survey. J Crit Care [Internet]. 2016;31(1):54–7. Available from:. https://doi.org/10.1016/j.jcrc.2015.09.032.

4. Remick DG, Xioa H. Hypothermia and sepsis. Front Biosci. 2006;11(1 P.889–1198):1006–13.

5. Wiewel MA, Harmon MB, van Vught LA, Scicluna BP, Hoogendijk AJ, Horn J, et al. Risk factors, host response and outcome of hypothermic sepsis. Crit Care [Internet]. 2016;20(1):1–9. Available from:. https://doi.org/10.1186/s13054-016-1510-3.

6. Rhodes A, Evans LE, Alhazzani W, Levy MM, Antonelli M, Ferrer R, et al. Surviving sepsis campaign: international guidelines for management of sepsis and septic shock: 2016. Crit Care Med. 2017;45:486–552.

7. Nishida O, Ogura H, Egi M, Fujishima S, Hayashi Y, Iba T, et al. The Japanese clinical practice guidelines for management of Sepsis and Septic Shock 2016 (J-SSCG 2016). J Intensive Care [Internet]. 2018;6:7. Available from: https://www.ncbi.nlm.nih.gov/pubmed/29435330

8. Cajander P, Edmark L, Ahlstrand R, Magnuson A, de Leon A. Effect of positive end-expiratory pressure on gastric insufflation during induction of anaesthesia when using pressure-controlled ventilation via a face mask: a randomised controlled trial. Eur J Anaesthesiol. 2019;36(9):625–32.

9. Higgs A, McGrath BA, Goddard C, Rangasami J, Suntharalingam G, Gale R, et al. Guidelines for the management of tracheal intubation in critically ill adults. Br J Anaesth [Internet]. 2018;120(2):323–52. Available from:. https://doi.org/10.1016/j.bja.2017.10.021.

10. Panzer O, Moitra V, Sladen RN. Oliver Panzer. Crit Care Clin [Internet]. 2009;25(3):451–69. Available from:. https://doi.org/10.1016/j.ccc.2009.04.004.

11. Stollings JL, Diedrich DA, Oyen LJ, Brown DR. Rapid-sequence intubation: a review of the process and considerations when choosing medications. Ann Pharmacother. 2014;48(1):62–76.

12. Colson JD. The pharmacology of sedation. Pain Physician. 2005;8(3):297–308.

13. Morris C, Perris A, Klein J, Mahoney P. Anaesthesia in haemodynamically compromised emergency patients: does ketamine represent the best choice of induction agent? Anaesthesia. 2009;64(5):532–9.

14. Gu WJ, Wang F, Tang L, Liu JC. Single-dose etomidate does not increase mortality in patients with sepsis: a systematic review

and meta-analysis of randomized controlled trials and observational studies. Chest. 2015;147(2):335–46.

15. Morris C, Perris A, Klein J, Mahoney P. Anaesthesia in haemodynamically compromised emergency patients: does ketamine represent the best choice of induction agent? Anaesthesia. 2009;64(5):532–9.

16. Chan CM, Mitchell AL, Shorr AF. Etomidate is associated with mortality and adrenal insufficiency in sepsis: a meta-analysis. Crit Care Med. 2012;40(11):2945–53. https://doi.org/10.1097/CCM.0b013e31825fec26;

17. Jabre P, Combes X, Lapostolle F, Dhaouadi M, Ricard-Hibon A, Vivien B, et al. Etomidate versus ketamine for rapid sequence intubation in acutely ill patients: a multicentre randomised controlled trial. Lancet. 2009;374(9686):293–300. https://doi.org/10.1016/S0140-6736(09)60949-1. Epub 2009 Jul 1;

18. Albert SG, Ariyan S, Rather A. The effect of etomidate on adrenal function in critical illness: a systematic review. Intensive Care Med. 2011;37(6):901–10. https://doi.org/10.1007/s00134-011-2160-1. Epub 2011 Mar 4;

19. Griesdale DEG. Etomidate for intubation of patients who have sepsis or septic shock – where do we go from here? Crit Care. 2012;16(6):6–7.

20. Edwin SB, Walker PL. Controversies surrounding the use of etomidate for rapid sequence intubation in patients with suspected sepsis. Ann Pharmacother. 2010;44(7–8):1307–13.

21. Ray DC, Mckeown DW. Effect of induction agent on vasopressor and steroid use, and outcome in patients with septic shock. Crit Care. 2007;11(3):1–8.

22. Wagner BKJ, O'Hara DA. Pharmacokinetics and pharmacodynamics of sedatives and analgesics in the treatment of agitated critically ill patients. Clin Pharmacokinet. 1997;33(6):426–53.

23. Ballow SL, Kaups KL, Anderson S, Chang M. A standardized rapid sequence intubation protocol facilitates airway management in critically injured patients. J Trauma Acute Care Surg. 2012;

24. Filanovsky Y, Miller P, Kao J. Myth: ketamine should not be used as an induction agent for intubation in patients with head injury. Can J Emerg Med. 2010;12(2):154–201.

25. Murray H, Marik PE. Etomidate for endotracheal intubation in sepsis: acknowledging the good while accepting the bad. Chest. 2005;127(3):707–9.

26. Simpson GD, Ross MJ, McKeown DW, Ray DC. Tracheal intubation in the critically ill: a multi-centre national study of practice and complications. Br J Anaesth [Internet]. 2012;108(5):792–9. Available from:. https://doi.org/10.1093/bja/aer504.

27. Gagnon DJ, Seder DB. Etomidate in sepsis: understanding the dilemma. J Thorac Dis. 2015;7(10):1699–701.

28. Langeron O, Cuvillon P, Ibanez-Esteve C, Lenfant F, Riou B, Le Manach Y. Prediction of difficult tracheal intubation: time for a paradigm change. Anesthesiology. 2012;117(6):1223–33. https://doi.org/10.1097/ALN.0b013e31827537cb;

29. Weingart SD, Levitan RM. Preoxygenation and prevention of desaturation during emergency airway management. Ann Emerg Med. 2012;59(3):165–75.e1. https://doi.org/10.1016/j.annemergmed.2011.10.002. Epub 2011 Nov 3;

30. Warters RD, Szabo TA, Spinale FG, Desantis SM, Reves JG. The effect of neuromuscular blockade on mask ventilation. Anaesthesia. 2011;66(3):163–7. https://doi.org/10.1111/j.1365-2044.2010.06601.x. Epub 2011 Jan 25;

31. Girard T. Pro: Rocuronium should replace succinylcholine for rapid sequence induction. Eur J Anaesthesiol. 2013;30(10):585–9. https://doi.org/10.1097/EJA.0b013e328363159a;

32. Marsch SC, Steiner L, Bucher E, Pargger H, Schumann M, Aebi T, et al. Succinylcholine versus rocuronium for rapid sequence intubation in intensive care: a prospective, randomized controlled trial. Crit Care. 2011 16;15(4):R199. https://doi.org/10.1186/cc10367;

33. Taha SK, El-Khatib MF, Baraka AS, Haidar YA, Abdallah FW, Zbeidy RA, et al. Effect of suxamethonium vs rocuronium on onset of oxygen desaturation during apnoea following rapid sequence induction: original article. Anaesthesia. 2010;65(4): p. 358–361;

34. McNamara MJ, Hardman JG. Hypoxaemia during open-airway apnoea: a computational modelling analysis. Anaesthesia. 2005;60(8):741–6. https://doi.org/10.1111/j.1365-2044.2005.04228.x;

35. Levitan R, Behringer E, Patel A. **Preoxygenation. In: Hagberg C, Artime C, Aziz M, editors. Benumof and Hagberg's airway management E-book. 4th ed: Elsevier Health Sciences; 2018. p. 16047–7280.

36. Patel A, Nouraei SAR. Transnasal humidified rapid-insufflation Ventilatory exchange (THRIVE): a physiological

method of increasing apnoea time in patients with difficult airways. Anaesthesia. 2015;70(3):323–9. https://doi.org/10.1111/anae.12923. Epub 2014 Nov 10;

37. Machlin HA, Myles PS, Berry CB, Butler PJ, Story DA, Heath BJ. End-tidal oxygen measurement compared with patient factor assessment for determining preoxygenation time. Anaesth Intensive Care. 1993;21(4):409-13;

38. Bhatia PK, Bhandari SC, Tulsiani KL, Kumar Y. End-tidal oxygraphy and safe duration of apnoea in young adults and elderly patients. Anaesthesia. 1997;52(2):175–8;

39. Benumof JL, Dagg R, Benumof R. Critical hemoglobin desaturation will occur before return to an unparalyzed state following 1 mg/kg intravenous succinylcholine. Anesthesiology. 1997;87:979–982;

40. Gambee AM, Hertzka RE, Fisher DM. Preoxygenation techniques: comparison of three minutes and four breaths. Anesth Analg. 1987;66(5):468–70

41. Farmery AD, Roe PG. A model to describe the rate of oxyhaemoglobin desaturation during apnoea. Br J Anaesth. 1996;76(2):284–91. https://doi.org/10.1093/bja/76.2.284;

Index

© Springer Nature Switzerland AG 2021   129
R. Garvin (ed.), *Intubating the Critically Ill Patient*,
https://doi.org/10.1007/978-3-030-56813-9

Printed in the United States
By Bookmasters